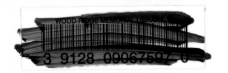
If

D1502656

If

A Mother's Memoir

LISE MARZOUK

Translated from the French by Adriana Hunter

OTHER PRESS
NEW YORK

Originally published in 2018 as Si by Éditions Gallimard, Paris

Production editor: Yvonne E. Cárdenas
Text Designer: Jennifer Daddio / Bookmark Design & Media Inc.
This book was set in Horley MT by Alpha Design & Composition
of Pittsfield, NH

1 3 5 7 9 10 8 6 4 2

Library of Congress Cataloging-in-Publication Data

Names: Revol-Marzouk, Lise, author. | Hunter, Adriana, translator.
Title: If : a mother's memoir / Lise Marzouk ; translated from the French
by Adriana Hunter.
Other titles: Si. English
Description: New York : Other Press, [2019] | Originally published as Si
(Paris : Gallimard, 2018).
Identifiers: LCCN 2019015345 | ISBN 9781590510971 (pbk.) |
ISBN 9781590510964 (ebook)
Subjects: LCSH: Revol-Marzouk, Lise. | Cancer in children—Patients—France—
Biography. | Cancer in children—Patients—France—Family relationships.
Classification: LCC RC281.C4 R4813 2019 | DDC 618.92/9940092 [B]—dc23
LC record available at https://lccn.loc.gov/2019015345

To Olivier

To my children

To the people who were there

If it were something in between, like
the gap between linden and laurel, in the garden,
like chill air on eyes and mouth
as you step, unthinking now, through your life,
if, yes, if it were just that footstep ventured
outside…
A subtle thought, but, should the fabric of the body tear,
what thought will stitch it back together?

—PHILIPPE JACCOTTET
À la lumière d'hiver

Give me back oh give me back my sky and my music

—LOUIS ARAGON
"Le Printemps" from Le Crève-coeur

Genesis

1

You're sitting on a rush-seat chair in the kitchen. You just turned ten. You have your mouth wide open and I'm exploring it.

The thing's abnormally large, I can see that. An incongruous, deformed irregular ball. It's taking up half the space, masking its twin in the background, pushing aside your uvula in the middle. What I'm really worried about are the black threads. They wriggle into the folds, like fuliginous rivulets streaming through valleys of pink flesh. Black is *not* physiological. My first fleeting thoughts and words. For now, these words play on a loop inside my skull. I can't break away from them. They cling to my mind just as these dark deposits cling to your tonsil. Viscous, cloying, repulsive. Black is not physiological. A stupid euphemism intended to postpone the terrible truth, which has already insinuated itself into me. And I know the facts: black flesh is decomposing flesh. The fetid breath you've been exhaling the last few days would be enough to convince me. We've laughed about that plenty. I'm not laughing now. I'm in no doubt: what I'm looking at is putrefying, with the color and smell of death.

Rational thinking comes trooping in like a detachment of guards. Or rather a militia. It forbids all prevarication, prescribes action, directing me to an internet page all about black throats, to find an acceptable answer. Not harmless but not unbearable. I scan quickly through the page, from one pathology to another. "Necrotic tonsillitis." Perfect. I've found my solution. The tonsil is dying. You, on the other hand, are fine. A quick excision and it will all be over. The rational dictatorship conjures up its guillotine. Elimination with no damage to the guilty party. Clack. Off to the clinic, clean job, no mess. In making this choice, the dictatorship rejected a long list of minor ills—short-lived infections and other consequences of poor hygiene—set out on the first half of the page, and thereby conceded a fragment of terrain to my premonition of horror. Peace of mind definitely warrants sacrificing one tiny organ. Because on the altar of this still-bleeding tonsil, to the benefit of this same offering, peace of mind managed to ignore the last lines on that page, although it glimpsed them, just enough to grasp their terrifying relevance. The enemy is in fact already there, skulking at the back of the platoon, and—behind its paradoxically sweet, resonant name—it trails a cortege of indescribable fears and sorrows, and tries to lure my mind into its vertiginous dance. I refuse to pronounce its name. Back to the middle of the page. "Necrotic tonsillitis."

Then come the decisions. It's midnight, you're tired, you're in your pajamas and ready to go back to bed. The painkiller has done its work, your throat doesn't hurt so much. The doctor on call will do. Better to avoid going to the hospital this evening. I call. Forty-five minutes elapse. You've gone back to sleep. The doctor shows up. Getting paunchy, shirt of dubious cleanliness, shapeless jacket, corduroy pants, worn leather briefcase. A few despicable social observations occur to me: poor-taste jokes about the sartorial and salary-related similarities between this night-duty GP and my fellow lecturers; an inadmissible contempt, distantly inherited from my family, for a man who most likely failed his residency thirty years ago, condemning himself to this job as an itinerant owl to top up his rather inglorious pay; and then a purely artistic interest in the varied prism around the contours of his eyes, the multicolored bags of a nocturnal rep for public health. Still, his homely appearance immediately gives me confidence. This is not the man to take us on down that internet page. We can rest easy. I can tell he's an expert in the flu, upset stomachs, measles, and other seasonal or childhood ailments. It only remains for me to coax him onto my terrain. Might as well come right out with it: "I think my son has necrotic tonsillitis. Well, you tell me, you know better than I do. One of his tonsils, but only one of them, is swollen and dark purple, almost black." Then it's repeat kitchen, repeat wide-open mouth, repeat flashlight, repeat teaspoon on tongue, repeat tonsil. "When will you ever stop opening your mouth?" I tease you with a smile. Oh my, aren't we having fun. We await the verdict, dimly anxious. "Ah yes, those black lines *are* strange"—you think so too, right—"it looks like tonsillitis but without the white spots"—there, now we're getting somewhere, that's reassuring—"it must be necrotic tonsillitis, it's nothing to worry about"—we did it. End of Act I.

Act II. But now, seriously, what should I do? Because I *did* read those lines at the bottom of the internet page. And I wouldn't want my delightful collaborator, devoted though he is to continued friendship between our respective corporations, to cause my son to run any risks. The ever-dependable rational militia sends me reinforcements. It has a secret weapon that means I can advance under cover. "Will he definitely need surgery? Because, you see, we're flying to Morocco in six days. Will he be fit to travel by next Saturday?" The journey angle is both real and irrefutable. Nothing quite like a deadline to get the wolf across the river. Handled correctly, the goat and the cabbage should also make the crossing unharmed. But Homely is an expert with more than one trick up his sleeve. And he categorically refuses to cross the Rubicon, let alone the Styx, with my whole menagerie. "Listen, we can't be sure, it might not need surgery at all. The best thing would be to go see an ENT specialist in town in two or three days to see how it's developing. Then you'll know where you stand for Morocco." Now, that I was not expecting. Back to the starting blocks. Unless...

I try a different tack. Tough luck for rational thinking and its troops. I open the door to the unexpected, just a fraction. I know for sure the conniving bastard, the enemy masked behind its honeyed little name will put its foot in there. If not a whole foot, at least the toes, a hint of it, the fear of it and the nagging thought of the possibility of it. But hey, we have to make the most of what's available. After all, this really matters, this is about my son. We can't always guarantee our own mental comfort. "You know, we nearly took him to the emergency room at Necker this evening, but then we thought that was over the top, maybe not necessary, maybe not the right thing." Homely doesn't see the trap. He falls into it like a greenhorn. "You know, they have a specialist ENT emergency department at Necker." No, I didn't know that, thanks. I do now. I also know the black river has just claimed its first victim.

Monday, December 17. Day One.

Carried by the combined energy of denial and hope, Lise continues to resist, for a while, just overnight. She swims against the current and keeps her head above water till dawn. But then it takes too much effort. There needs to be some pretense of hesitation, a few invented digressions: the analysis lab to carry out the blood count prescribed last night, the café on the corner to avoid going hungry, a few calls to cancel the day's appointments. Meanwhile the anxiety builds. It swells and fattens in step with the tonsil that has doubled in size in the space of a few hours, forming a small protuberance visible to the naked eye on the child's neck, just below the ear. And, in Lise's mind, the sight of it is reinforced by echoes of the words she glimpsed the night before, this image and those words corresponding with sickening insistence. This tide of anxiety would inevitably scoop her up eventually—dragging her in its backwash, its endless waves clutching and then releasing her—were it not held back by her husband's conspicuous innocence. Olivier, it seems, saw nothing, heard nothing, and intuited nothing in all this but the strategies of a rational mind. He willingly slipped into a silent, sterilized neutral space, cradled in potential regret for a sun-kissed trip condemned by a stupid winter infection. And Lise didn't have the heart to wrench him from his haven and forcibly make him listen to the words she had read, and see the things written under those words. Perhaps—out of love, respect, or reticence—she hoped this would spare him, would avoid drawing him into her wake. Perhaps it suits her just fine to have an innocent by her side, someone whose delicious ingenuousness can prolong this "before" phase that she can tell will soon be over. Perhaps she's also afraid he won't have the strength to cope, he'll be overwhelmed all too soon, meaning she'll need to save not just one but two of her crew. Perhaps she has already assessed that she won't have what it takes to do this, that she would have to choose, and the choice is a foregone conclusion. Perhaps this is the real reason she tells Olivier nothing: she doesn't want to leave him to be mangled on the reefs and to run aground, abandoned and inert on the shore. They must each fight their own

*fight, with their own weapons and at their own speed, she gets
that already. So Lise decides to go to Necker and Olivier drives.*

I'm slightly reassured when we get to the emergency room.
At first. It has the advantage of instantly drowning our isolation in a hubbub of cries, coughs, expectorations, and other
excretions. We're no longer alone, that's for sure. Besides,
the charming young man on reception told us with great
aplomb that the visible black threads in your throat must be
deposits of blood, residues of a harmless infection. The fact
he hadn't examined the tonsil and had absolutely no compe-
tence to evaluate it doesn't matter much: we're not going to
deny ourselves a few extra minutes of immunity. Cocooned
in our illusory confidence, we're now eyeing the snotty spec-
imens around us with all the arrogance of monarchs spared
by common afflictions. Still, it's only a brief respite, too brief
not to be suspect. A doctor calls us. He is short, dark-haired,
overworked-looking. He puts us in a cubicle. "Doctor
G...," he announces—an inarticulate and incomprehensible name—"don't move, I'll be back." A pause. And off
we go again: the unexplained tiredness, the abnormal tonsil,
the smelly deposits, the inconclusive duty doctor, the hopes
for Morocco. Here you are again, sitting with your mouth
open and your tonsil laid bare. The thing's grown so huge
that you struggle to widen your jaws. The vestiges of fresh,

pink healthy flesh have now almost completely disappeared under the magma of purplish black, like a sea urchin's orangey gonads buried in the fetid scramble of its digestive, circulatory, and nervous systems. Dr. G stands up and takes a moment. I swear he's paled. Nothing else is said, but this pallor, coupled with the momentary hiatus, speaks volumes. It nudges my vigilance to maximum alert. I didn't get his name, but I know Dr. G's every breath, every look, every move, every emotion. First a change of pace. After the suspense, now the race. A sudden about-turn, a nervy, active quickening step, jerking movements, halting breath. A new rhythm, soon hammered out loudly as a leitmotif—"okay, no time to lose"—whose convulsive, almost spasming repetition strains the whole room, makes the air unbreathable, sucks out all the oxygen, as if the ER's heart were accelerating furiously, signaling an imminent cardiac arrest. Hardly surprising then, in the circumstances, that Dr. G goes for reinforcements. He hurries back accompanied by an intern. And now the two of them come to a standstill a couple of yards from us, and they hover there, frozen, looking at each other, solemn-faced, heads tilted, contemplative as the peasants in Millet's *Angelus*. Except that they're not praying to some all-merciful God, but quietly exchanging a few unspeakable words. No, this definitely isn't *The Angelus*. In this little booth, on this particular morning, it's much more like a death knell that's sounding, in secret, for me alone. Because, inaudible though it may be, I hear what Dr. G whispers in his coworker's ear. Not all of it, not in detail, but enough. Just two words, in fact. But not any old words. And now I know. I don't believe it, but I know.

Stage two. That's what my ear alighted on. *Stage 2?* Wasn't that a sports TV show my family used to watch back in the seventies? I wish these words would transport me somewhere else, to my childhood and the days when I lay on the carpet and—hoping in vain to join my unreachable siblings—forced myself to be crazy about the sports news, to sing along to their team's anthem, rail at ill-judged corners, and moan about bribed refs. *Stage 2*, the hand on a stopwatch ticking off the seconds and cross-fading to a sprinter, a cyclist, a discus-thrower, a ball. *Stage 2*, mustard yellow letters in relief against a red background. *Stage 2* with its magical, captivating title sequence. Oh, how I'd love to vault onboard the imaginary world evoked by that name, and launch freely between the gods of the pitch and the other cathodic cults of the time, all those barely remembered dramas and game shows, and that Sunday mass broadcast. Shows as old as I am, fragments of media eternity.

But I inherited more than this televisual culture from my childhood. My original language comprised a quite different vocabulary that suddenly seems to be tragically incarnated in this emergency room at Necker Hospital. A vocabulary installed even before my birth, experienced through the cancer that affected my father at the age of thirty-three, endorsed by that same father's disabled status brought home from the Algerian war of independence, transmuted by the accident that cost my brother an eye the year he turned nine, crystalized in the family's taboo illnesses (Alzheimer's in the maternal grandfather I never knew, depression in one aunt and psychosis in another), and the whole lot distilled and absorbed in utero during the hours on the analyst's couch that worked up toward my unplanned conception, then endured throughout my father's crippling neurosis paired with my mother's depression that marked my arrival and lasted through my childhood. Yes, that's my inheritance: an infinite lexical landscape of physical and mental suffering, a fertile terrain of every malfunction, a terrain my forebears were careful to master and tend, probably for fear of being identified merely as sharecroppers. Austere biologist ancestors; parents who specialized in the brain in every condition—a psychiatrist father and a pediatric neurologist mother; and finally, my sister and brothers who followed in these parental footsteps with remarkable oedipal constancy: the first son is a pediatrician like Mommy, the daughter a psychiatrist like Daddy, and the younger brother, attempting a commendable deviation, a psycho-motor therapist.

I know about "stage two." The last and late-born offspring of this unusual dynasty, I had to learn this strange language if I was to escape the cavernous solitude to which it relegated me. What with the tyrannical silence of an apartment that morphed into a doctor's office during the

day with its living room–cum–consulting room and its dining room–cum–waiting room, a place where the scantest
conversation was spilt hastily in the break between two patients, and, come the evening, the sudden invasion of this
same space by emphatic accounts of catastrophes glimpsed
at the hospital, there was no room for other words, about
school, friendships, the trifling but vital pains and struggles of early childhood—my words. "Stage two," then.
Sadly, I knew what that meant way too early.

I then did everything I could to erase this vocabulary
from my memory. First, I chose a different professional
route, one that focused on words, in fact, in the hope that
I could then build my own idiom and escape this official
language. By a delightful irony of fate, I emerged a doctor.
Then I married. On the very day of our wedding, my father-
in-law accidently electrocuted himself, wedding canceled, a
month in a coma, years of physiotherapy, some incurable
after-effects. Then I had my first child. Suspected coma at
birth, sudden death avoided by the skin of our teeth in his
first week. I'm not even counting the miscarriages, they're
too commonplace, even late ones, nor the autoimmune condition that struck during my thirties and at least has the
tact to be unidentified and unnamed. In short, years spent
playing hide-and-seek with this weighty heritage, skipping
between my analyst's couch and the arts, to preserve you,
my children, from its morbid legacy. And now look where
we are, ten days after your tenth birthday.

"Stage two." I get it. I know what's wrong with you, know its name, and I also know that this "two" can grow faster even than your tonsil, with each increment narrowing your chances. I look up, mentally stepping in time with Dr. G; I in turn go pale and start privately intoning the day's leitmotif: "Okay, no time to lose."

"We're going to take a biopsy." Could the young intern have the impudence to think that, sheltered behind this technical term, he's not in the line of fire? I'll give him a taste of these sidestepping tactics. "Why a biopsy?" A moment's hesitation—it seems he never came across this question in his multiple-choice exams—then, improvising clumsily and with feigned detachment: "Oh, you know, sometimes some bacteria can't be detected without one." "But I would have thought," I plow on, "that biopsies aren't used *only* for identifying bacteria." A filter of dread in his eyes, his features chalkier than ever, his head swinging repeatedly from left to right, where on earth has Dr. G gone? Yes, quick, a doctor, the intern's about to pass out. I won't get anything more from him, that's for sure. And so I spare him, particularly as the procedure, which is painful, makes you howl. I have better things to do than torture this poor boy. And while I'm consoling you, Dr. G does return. No more games. "I can guess what you're looking for with this biopsy, Doctor. When will we have the results?" "In two days, on Wednesday." And then a little sentence, a harmless but at the same time devastating comment. A combination of simple words that opens the door to chaos, ten blows dealt to the normal working order of our existence: "For your trip to Morocco, maybe check the cancelation terms."

What is said in the car on the way home from the hospital, no one remembers. They probably each pursue their own logic: One thinking about the insurance for the flights, the second about the imminent catastrophe, the third about his pain. Three solitary paths and yet they converge, meet, and become intertwined in a few witty, tender, or comforting words. Three solitary paths straining to link up with the afternoon's schedule, the solid structure of everyday life. In these moments deleted from their memories, it is agreed that the mother and child will spend the rest of the day together, the child won't go to school. The reasons for this decision also differ in each of their minds: compensating for the morning's torments, preparing to confront the worst, an unhoped-for opportunity to skip lessons. Curled up together with the living room blinds half lowered and a blanket over their feet, Lise and her son prepare to watch a movie while Olivier heads back to work. The child has been allowed to decide everything, as if, on the threshold of total constraint, he must be granted this fragment of freedom. How they sit, the choice of film, dubbed as opposed to subtitled, it's all down to him. So, it's Star Wars *then. In French, the first educationally retrograde step taken in the name of his illness.* Star Wars, *the film that this eldest child,*

condemned by his younger siblings to endless reiterations of car-
toons, is always asking to watch from the full height of his ten
years. Star Wars, prefiguring the battle they will soon have to
wage together. Two hours of movie, time suspended, with Lise
fluctuating between abandoning herself to fiction and returning
to reality, using the excuse of the darker scenes to put her arms
around her child, whose life she suddenly realizes is so fragile. It
also occurs to her that when the film is over it will be time to pick
up the results of the blood count taken that morning, time to ask
the first questions and cope with the first answers. Just a few
minutes more, a pointless moratorium. The child can stay alone
after this, he's fine. It isn't far to the lab: you need only walk up
rue Claude-Bernard, the very street, although Lise doesn't yet
know this, that will lead her and Olivier to the Curie Institute
for many months, every day and every night, to see what the
illness and the treatments have left of their son.

But on this Monday her destiny doesn't take her to the end
of the street, to bear right down rue d'Ulm and then left into
rue Louis-Thuillier. For now she stops halfway. The trip is long
enough, though, for her to call one of her brothers. The eldest
in the family, a pediatrician of some note, with a smile cour-
tesy of "Émail diamant" toothpaste and the requisite empathy
and narcissism. The conversation is short: "I'm calling because
I think my boy has cancer." The big brother to the rescue smiles,
suspects exaggeration, then reassures. Lise summarizes: black
tonsil, stage two, biopsy. The doctor prevaricates. Cancer, well,
maybe. She must get these results. It's not complicated: if the

blood counts are good, no point waiting till Wednesday, her
mind will be at rest this evening. If not . . . Hundreds of yards
uphill covered at a run, the envelope ripped open as soon as she's
out of the lab, tears in her eyes, her hands shaking, as she comes
back down the street. On the left, in black, the child's figures.
On the right, in blue, the norms, a minimum-maximum range.
A sinister abstract of his future in a cryptic alphabet: g, %, μl,
mm³. Lise reads, compares, rereads, compares, rereads again.
Perfect results. They're saved. There's nothing wrong with him.

Back at home I collapse, curling up tightly on the sofa. Even
though the adventure ended well, it turned against me. It
clearly illustrates the side effects of a mistrustful imagination forever in thrall to its medical inheritance. I draw my
own conclusions from it, radical ones of course, and make
resolutions, resolutely firm ones. Always. I take pleasure in
playing back the different scenes in which I went astray,
revisit the crossroads where my mind took a wrong turn. I
dismantle the mechanisms of my digression, reformulating
a meaning compatible with the biological results. I emerge
from this exhausted, but profoundly relieved. That is when
the phone rings. "Mrs. M, this is Doctor G. Is your husband
home?" "Not yet." "Are you alone?" "Yes, with the children." The exchange is brief, the words elliptical. "I'm so
sorry, Mrs. M, we'd never normally say this over the phone,

but we have to in this case. It's the only oncological emergency in a child. The biopsy is not good. You need to come back in this evening, right away, to Necker, your son starts chemotherapy at the Curie Institute tomorrow. Your husband already knows, I just called him in his car, he's nearly home." I say nothing, or almost. "Okay, I understand. Just one question: Does my son have time to eat before going back to Necker?" "Yes, well, don't waste too much time. Good luck to you. Goodbye." I hang up. And sit on the floor. And see myself sitting on the floor. And see myself seeing myself sitting on the floor. Not because I need to, but out of mimicry. Because I remember that in bad films people do this in life's crises. I become two people so I can incarnate the lamenting mother. But I'm back on my feet soon enough. To be honest, I have no reason to be on the floor. My legs haven't buckled under me and my head isn't spinning. I don't even feel surprised. I'm an athlete exquisitely trained for impending catastrophe. I'm permanently waiting for it. Always have been, since I began. And having trodden and retrodden this path today has greatly increased my grounding and concentrated my strength. I simply feel I've come to the beginning of the road. And I think starkly, *Right, this is it.* Just then a key turns in the lock and Olivier comes in. Hi. Kisses, smiles, perfunctory versions of them. "I've just had Doctor G on the phone. Have you heard?" "Yes, he called me on my way home." I feel sorry for Olivier. It must have been appalling hearing about it in those circumstances. On the road, trapped in a metal box, halfway across town, in among the traffic, and strangers. I can picture him at the wheel. "Mr. M, this is Doctor G, are you driving? You should pull over." Hell on earth. I was lucky. I was on familiar, intimate territory, close to you. I could admire you in the flesh. I could substitute the fresh invigorating sight of you for those savage words. I could go into your room, talk to you, touch you, smile at you. And fill the crevasse of your future absence with the you who is here now. Anyway, it's done. The news has been given to the mother. And it has been given to the father. This pivotal information, that is constructing a before and an after, founding a new chaotic order on the ruins, is something that we, your parents, did not share, either in form or in content. Will we manage to stay united in the battle despite this fundamental schism? I can only obscurely gauge the consequences. I have better things to think about. Come on, no time to lose. First, get you to accept that we need to go back to the hospital for more tests. Allow me to introduce lying, by omission. Second, find someone to look after your brother and sister. Third, avoid making a big deal of this, in what we say, how we move, how we look at each other, how we breathe. We'll make you laugh, a little, on the way back to Necker, a twilight trip completing the hazardous circle embarked on in the morning.

———

What happens on that Monday evening and the ensuing night will soon be a fathomless gulf in Lise's memory. She will become aware of this defect only four days later during her first appointment with a psychiatrist at the Curie Institute who invites her to describe the early stages of the child's illness. She will have no trouble listing the first signs, will even enjoy it, going into details, emphasizing the paradoxes, making the occasional ironic comment, exultant to be doing so well and showing such strength as she copes with the abomination meted out to her. But to her complete astonishment she will have to stop dead halfway through a sentence. Pulled up short in her flow of words, reduced to silence, abandoned and helpless, robbed of any logic or chronology. Deprived of words, images, sounds, and feelings. Empty. "So, we got to Necker and then . . . then . . . then—that's really scary, I have no idea." A frightening and fascinating sensation she's never had before. Ricocheting the same word as it bounces off the surface of her memories but fails to make its way in, regrouping with a brief ellipsis before coming up against silence all over again. A complete failure to get a grip on her own story, the inescapable disappearance of part of herself. Twenty-four hours erased by the violence of this trauma. "But what the hell did we do when we got to Necker?" It will take Lise weeks to piece together the events, only partially, then years to complete the narrative, joining the dots, filling the gaps with borrowings from other people's more reliable memories—meaning she had to question witnesses.

At about eight o'clock, so less than forty-five minutes since the phone call, the parents and child arrive outside the hospital. They pass the gatehouse at the main entrance and start looking for the building with the inscription "Emergencies" on it in red letters, find a parking space, then walk through a variety of doors: sliding doors, glass doors, fire doors, doors with port-hole windows. A difficult journey, undertaken almost without breathing, in the certainty that things will be better afterward, once Dr. G and his team take charge of them, support, inform, and even reassure them. When the last door is closed they set off down a long corridor. Listless light from sickly neon strips, lino-leum tiles on the floor, worn bench seats on the right, reception desk on the left. And no one. No one. How long exactly do they stay here like this, pacing up and down the corridor, exploring the succession of solitary, unlit closed rooms? Figures drifting in a ghost space. How long do they stay sitting on the worn seats, stifling their escalating anxiety with jokes? Someone does even-tually appear behind the desk. Who he is exactly, what his job might be, no one will ever know: night watchman, administra-tor, assistant nurse, certainly not a doctor. He asks their names, their address, some further information, and informs them that a nurse will come to set up a drip. Then time dilates again during another terrifying, sinister wait. It all feels so unreal that for a long while to come Lise and Olivier will wonder whether they really did see someone they knew in that deserted corridor, at this peculiar time in their lives. Whether Catherine, a single mother of two adopted children who attend the same school as *theirs, really did appear through the door with the porthole window and come to sit next to Lise. Catherine whom they have so often pitied for her tough unrelenting life torn between grueling work and family issues, Catherine, a Mother Courage buttressing her eldest child destroyed by abandonment, Catherine who this evening is nevertheless, at last, the lucky mother, because she's here for a simple ear infection. A contradictory coincidence: however familiar she may be, they can't say a word to this one other person present. Then Catherine leaves, the ear infection treated. And now, in this breeding ground of shadows, loneliness, and silence, fear is free to escalate. They each busy themselves. Olivier reads, the child plays, Lise takes pictures of him with her cell. An automatic activity, but one surreptitiously paired with the embryo of an unbearable thought: what if it's the last. The last image of his thick hair, the last sight of his plump peach complexion, the last proof that he lived healthily. This thought is aborted by the welcome but shamefully delayed arrival of a nurse. Or rather a student nurse. "I'm going to put him on a drip." "Why?" "I don't know, I was just told to put him on a drip." "And then what?" "I don't know, I was just told to put him on a drip." The student nurse doesn't know much. To tell the truth, she doesn't even know how to set up a drip. She pricks the needle into the child a first time, shaking, misses the vein, tries again, misses again, repeats her performance. Each failure makes her more unsure of herself, further reducing her already slender aptitude. Little bruises appear, everywhere, on the back of his hand. She's exhausted the area, looks for another, virgin*

*territory, near the wrist. She starts to panic, palpably. She has
tears in her eyes. She's pricked his skin to no avail ten times now.
"I can't do it. He doesn't have good veins. They keep slipping
under my fingers." Well, it does have to be somebody's fault.
Her stress eventually gets to the child. He cries, screams, wails.
"It hurts too much, Mommy, I'll never make it." His choice of
words lacerates his parents' hearts. If he only knew what lay
ahead. Actually, what does lie ahead? Who knows? Will there
finally be someone to tell them?*

The failed drip is too much for me. I need to get out. I thread
my way back through the doors, looking for the exit. Once
outside, I have to crouch down. This time it's very real.
My legs give way and I'm dizzy. I'm thwarted by having no
one to talk to. An absence that amputates me of all hope,
and horror grafts itself in its place. My thoughts break away
from me, scattering in myriad uncontrollable images and
ideas. A monster takes shape. It has a huge hideous head. Its
gaping distorted mouth keeps screaming, "It's the only oncological emergency for children." Counterfeiting my medical inheritance, this collection of words finds a diagnosis to
match it: acute aggressive leukemia. The sort that snatches
away a life in the space of a few days. Then the monster
uncoils its tentacles of terror and helplessness. I won't let
you die alone, in the hospital. We're going to set off, the two

of us, to climb the tallest, most magnificent mountain, and from there, from the perennial snows of its summit, we'll jump into the void together. A beautiful end. What about Anna? And Nils? Change the points on that railway track. I can't leave your brother and sister. My darling, I love you forever. I'll be by your side. I'll give you everything, everything, so there can be no regrets. But at the end, I'll have to stay behind. Will I have only two children then? An unbearable thought. No, there'll be three of you till the day I die. A proper family. You'll never be its phantom member. Your absence will underline how impossible it is to exist without you. I picture my mutilated world, the truncated pleasures, the excised laughter. A whole make-believe life bandaged over a gaping wound. The possibility of giving up blows over me like a wind. I turn my back to it. I won't let the monster devour me. I need help. I need to talk to someone. I take out my cell and call my mother. The time has come to tell my loved ones.

"Mom, it's Lise. I have bad news. My big boy has cancer. I forbid you to cry in front of me." At this exact moment, even though it still seems this cancer might destroy my entire life, it begins a clandestine reconstruction process. It has just taught me to reject empathy and pathos. It has just taught me that, to be the best mother I can be to my son, I need to stop being one to my mother. Because I have decided, almost subconsciously, to apply the logic of concentric circles, fine-tuned and tested during previous crises in our lives. Every calamity is like the ripples formed on the surface by a stone thrown into water. The closer these ripples are to the center, the deeper and more pronounced they are. As they get further away, they are less defined and more spaced apart. And this implies a direction of travel. Each circle must be able to lean on the next, without reciprocation. You are at the center, the most affected. You will not bear our pain as parents. Neither will your brother and sister, in the second circle. Just as we, in the third circle, will not bear your grandparents' pain, or our friends', and they in turn must find support on which to draw strength, they must find people further removed from you. And so on till the last, almost imperceptible wrinkle. I remember nothing about my parents' reaction, other than that it is dignified and matches my hopes. The news has been imparted, once and for all. Now practical decisions can be addressed swiftly. "Would you like us to come to be with you? We could catch the last high-speed train from Bordeaux." "Yes, maybe, so you can look after the other two while I'm not there." "Your sister just happens to be heading for Paris for a colloquium. Do you want us to tell her?" "Yes, why not. She's a doctor, she could help us. Let's keep each other in the loop." I hang up. I breathe. I can go back in.

The waiting starts again, in a cubicle this time, with you lying down, a needle in your wrist. You've just come up from the hospital's basement, where they had to take you after the fiasco with the nurse, to put in the drip under anesthetic. A laughing gas mask, a few hallucinatory comments, and the job is done. Oh, how we'd laugh about your wild imaginings under the effects of nitrous oxide. But, truth be told, no one's laughing, especially not you: you're ashen, nauseous, and already exhausted. Someone walks past in the corridor, at last. I rush out. It's a woman, the duty intern. I frantically ask my first questions. I don't remember what they are. Neither can I remember her replies. She leaves. More waiting. Then another person comes. A doctor. He's young, not very tall, blue-eyed. He looks the straight-talking type. "Can I have a word, Doctor?" He takes me aside, to a room with windows, probably the nurses' office. He closes the door, perches on the edge of the table, facing me. He maintains eye contact. I trust him. "Does anyone know what's wrong with my son?" "We don't yet have definitive results from the biopsy, but it's a lymphoma or a type of leukemia." The word hurts. What if? What if I was right in my incoherent raving? The only oncological emergency for children. "Will he die?" The question pops out, of its own accord. I need to know. "Look, I wouldn't have said it so bluntly a few years ago, but there are now treatments. The Curie Institute knows how to tackle these conditions. Of course it will take a long time and it will be difficult. And there are no guarantees, particularly as we're still waiting for a precise diagnosis. But they know how to tackle them." His words are both hard and soothing. "For now, we'll keep your son in overnight. We'll scan him and give him a first treatment via the drip. He'll go to the Curie tomorrow to start chemotherapy." "One last question, Doctor: What should I tell my son?" "Well, tell him his blood is sick, and that's why we have to inject stuff into his blood." I like this. It's logical and clear. I'll use it. "Thank you, Doctor, thank you." When I come out of the room I go over to Olivier. We haven't yet spoken to each other this evening. I tell him about my conversation, take him in my arms, and say we're going to get through this, together. I don't believe it. I say it simply because I'd like him to say it to me.

My phone rings. My sister, Mathilde, is in the hospital's upper floors looking for us. She arrives two minutes later, trailing her suitcase and grumbling. "I thought he was up there, no one told me." Paradoxically, her bad mood cheers me up. Familiar territory at last. And I know that with her there won't be even a whiff of pathos. But most of all, she's here. I cling once more to the muddle-headed hope that something is being mended here by grace of this catastrophe. Something that draws on my painful roots. Mathilde, I've been told, experienced my birth—the year she turned eleven—as a criminal invasion, and didn't talk to my mother for many months. A result of her life up until then, which was most likely as damaging as mine. And our inevitably chaotic relationship is built on this unstable foundation. My parents chose her as my godmother, thinking this would help her invest emotionally in someone she didn't want. And there have been signs of that at various key moments in my life. A sort of silent intensity that occasionally displayed affection for me. But there was also, predominantly, its opposite. A lack of thoughtfulness, withdrawals, stinging rejections, instead of an affinity rich with promise. Mathilde didn't have the words. And I, being too young, always found them too late. I had to grow up with this deficiency, with the deep-seated conviction that, although I wasn't really sure why, I intrinsically deserved the cruel privations of what I was given. Until that fateful day in 2003. My mother's seventieth birthday. My brothers had given me the job of finding a present for my mother from the four of us, but my sister didn't like the idea. This difference of opinion fanned the flames of her ancient jealousy. She became barbaric. A few—hideous—words screeched into the phone. "No one in the family likes you, anyway. You're hardly even human. Your life's an insult to the lives of patients I treat in my clinic every day. One day you'll hit absolute rock bottom, and then you'll get it." I didn't know how to respond, and did, in fact, end up hitting rock bottom. Although I didn't understand any of it.

This evening, eight years later, in this hospital, when my son has a potentially fatal illness, do I finally have the right to claim to be human? Can I finally, thanks to my newfound complicity with the dying, accord myself legitimacy to exist? It's a strong possibility, because, in the name of this crisis, the sisterly authority is granting me some remission and is honoring me with her presence. The despicable calculations of a macabre bookkeeper: buying myself a crumb of clemency over my son's weakening body. The worst of it is I'm instantly taken in by this wily deal. The worst of it is the horror in front of me now is so bad that only this petty fixer-upper trade-off makes it bearable. A tidy little arrangement with death. At the expense of my dignity perhaps, but what does that matter. I have much more important things to worry about.

The rest of the evening goes astonishingly well. Lise, Olivier, and their son embark on an active phase. Doing something means they can stop thinking. Not thinking means they can do something. Added to this is a productive form of curiosity. Everything is a distraction, an entertainment even, and overrides the tragedy. First, they need to go downstairs to the scanner. A wheelchair is supplied for the child, who sits in it without any fuss. Once in the basement, the nocturnal calm becomes a blessing: the parents and child launch themselves down the deserted corridors at breakneck speed, taking turns to push each other in the chair, cornering tightly, rolling on the floor breathless and smiling at the end of their mad dash. Childhood reclaims its rights. Next comes the preparation procedure for the scanner, another form of entertainment with actors, technicians, costumes, props, and endlessly rehearsed moves. Lise puts on the lead apron, pretends to crumple under its weight.

The child laughs out loud. And his laugh has no trouble penetrating the lead, electrifying his mother to the core. Galvanized, she repeats the performance. A running gag. She'd do
anything to ensure her son keeps lighting up like this. And
what she does and says is complete nonsense, an outpouring of
witticisms, jokes, and winks, finding everything amusing for
his amusement. Nothing can suppress fate, Lise knows that.
So she might as well play along. Of course, the questions are
still there, torturing her very flesh at every possible occasion,
stinging her in the briefest interlude. The time the child spends
in the scanner is an opportunity to put these questions to her
sister and the medical staff. They remain unanswered. It's far
too soon for answers. Too soon, in fact, even for questions. It
won't be until the child is transferred to the Curie, tomorrow,
that his parents see an oncologist. For now, they go back up-
stairs. A bed in a twin room, the adults wait in the corridor.
Wait for what, exactly? Nothing in particular. For time to
pass, for this tomorrow to come. The waiting is filled with silences, cigarettes, inconsequential exchanges, even jokes. The
husband and wife look at each other, the sisters approach each
other cautiously, tenderness blooms, but unvoiced. At three in
the morning, with the child finally asleep, Mathilde leaves for
her hotel and Lise goes home while Olivier starts the first of a
long series of nights on a camp bed at his son's feet.

When Lise comes home at 3:30 a.m., she finds her mother
in her bed. It feels terribly incongruous. Particularly as her
father is asleep in her hospitalized child's empty bed. She

understands that this is a self-defense reflex in the face of their distress. Some people hold each other close, others hold each other in bed. It's just unexpected for a woman not well versed in signs of maternal affection. In all honesty, Lise isn't entirely sure this is to do with protecting and consoling her. She can't help thinking it might be geared instead toward the reciprocal. One thing she does know for sure, though, is that she has no desire to spend the rest of the night next to her mother. And she says so. She needs to refuel her batteries. In the morning she'll have to deal with the younger children's school, the look in people's eyes, settling her boy at the Curie, and the start of chemotherapy. The time has come to arm herself. She takes half an Atarax and collapses, shattered, into a soupy lethargy.

It's a harsh wake-up. Submerged within the folds of artificial sleep, her head weighs heavy. Her eyelids are taut, her neck stiff. No part of her has so much as quivered before the images come crashing in, anarchic and lapidary. And the images are paired with a riot of words. Relentless reminiscences of the night before. A shred of hope emerges from their very confusion. It takes the hypothetical form of a nightmare. For a moment, Lise finds herself assessing proof of this in the very onslaught and extravagance of her memories. Besides, her current circumstances also seem to support this possibility. The sheets are all messed up, aren't they? And she's covered *in sweat and her limbs are stiff. In the half-consciousness of morning on the day after the catastrophe, the boundary between illusion and reality reveals just how permeable it is. The dazed mother can see a way out because, having spent so much time thinking life was just a dream, she is now allowed to believe the horror was a hallucination. It doesn't strike her as totally impossible, although increasingly improbable. With each passing minute, signs for the case against do indeed accumulate. With her mind now awake, her memory recovers its acuity and reconstitutes a rigorous chronology of events. Their sheer length and orderliness point to reality. And are soon seconded by sensations: her hand reaching to find that Olivier isn't on the right-hand side of the bed, her mouth woolly from the Atarax, the tension gripping her breastbone. Reason fights on, searching for and finding explanations. Perhaps her husband went to work early, last night's supper didn't go down very well and she spent a restless night full of gloomy dreams. At last her eyes open and, on the chair by the bed, alight on the ultimate proof: a bag, her mother's bag. There's no room for doubt. All of it is— incontrovertibly, inescapably, mercilessly—true. She needs to get up and go into battle.*

2

I'm obsessed with the thought of your transfer to the Curie Institute. I'm to be there waiting for you at the end of the morning. But first I must honor my other life, the one I had before, the one involving your brother and sister, along with school, activities, friends, and the neighborhood. A life that will and must keep going. So this is what it means to have a sick child. Leading a double life, juggling the ordinary and the extraordinary, normality and anarchy. An irony of this fate is that it is my everyday life that becomes secondary, while the other life, the intruder, the parasite, becomes central, unabating, omnipotent, sucking the blood out of my physical, mental, and social space. When I'm on the street, in shops, in a café or out for dinner, I'll have to cheat the whole time in order not to stop being the woman I still was less than twenty-four hours ago. Becoming an actress playing the part of me, and putting on the mask of who I was. The character is more real than I am, a me that was once very much here, but is now lost. I must hide, if not the fact of the cancer itself, at least the deep fault line it has carved. Smiling, as usual. Listening, as usual. Understanding, as usual. And it starts right now, because I need to take Anna and Nils to school. I'll see so many friends and acquaintances who don't know. Their cheerful hellos will whip my face. How will I reply to the routine "How are you?" except with another "Fine, how are you?" only it will be more pointless and untruthful than ever. I don't even have to wait until then to come up with my performance. Getting out of bed, having breakfast, and preparing to leave stand in as a dress rehearsal. Now is the time to gauge the true— and incalculable—value of having your grandparents here. They help me turn the obstructed cogs of routine. Your grandmother serves breakfast while your grandfather gets Nils dressed. I don't yet have enough information to know what to say to the children, and I don't want to lie to them. And so I concentrate on what needs doing: tidying up, organizing school bags, and making after-school snacks. I'm longing for midday, and nothing else.

I don't know how I come to find myself sitting at a café table, on the corner of the street where the elementary school is. I must, at some point, have come out of the apartment building with the children, let them run along the charming passageway lined with artists' studios that leads to the rue Broca, walked under Port-Royal Bridge and up the rue des Lyonnais, gone into the nursery school, climbed the stairs to the third floor and left Nils with his teacher, not without explaining the situation in a few simple words, to preempt any possible distress in my little youngest. I must then have gone back downstairs, come out of the nursery school, continued up the rue des Lyonnais, and cut across toward the rue de l'Arbalète, where, in between the two schools, I would have seen dozens of familiar faces to whom I said nothing, before dropping Anna at the elementary school, not without explaining the situation in a few simple words to the head teacher to preempt any possible distress in my little middle child. I must have done all this, but so mechanically that I can't seem to remember it. Habit backed up by willpower. And now here I am, as usual in the Café d'Avant—the "Before" Café—whose name suddenly seems peculiarly preordained. And this will in fact be the place I come to unfailingly every morning for months on end, to spend half an hour breathing the air of my former social life, before going to take over from your father and staying at the Institute from 9 a.m. to 9 p.m.

This morning is different, though. I'm not sitting with the whole of the usual group of friends for a bit of idle chitchat. I'm at a separate table with my parents and two close friends. When did I tell them? Just now, when I came in, right after saying hello? Yesterday evening by text? I don't remember. It must have been a terrible shock; they have tears in their eyes. Not me. We're talking about you, slightly embarrassed, them because they don't know what to say, me because I can tell they're embarrassed. I hate

myself for denting the peace of their well-balanced lives
with my little personal catastrophe. I already experience
your illness as a weight threatening to destabilize the system that regulates our get-togethers here, a system based
on the blithe pleasure of superficial acquaintance. I can already feel the rift opening. My friends are quick to go join
the other group, as much of a relief for me as for them. My
mother goes to make a phone call. A few minutes later, a
man enters the café, comes over to me with a resolute step,
and hands me a business card. "We know each other by
sight, my wife's a doctor. I know a lot of people in oncology.
I know you're being sent to the Curie, but you must go to
Gustave Roussy, it's the best. Get in touch with Profes-
sor X, he's a pro." I rage internally. How can this stranger
appropriate this confidential, embryonic situation? What
does he think he knows about my son's illness, when I don't
know anything about it myself yet? And by what right is
he questioning the one solid thing that I have: the Curie
Institute, which, as well as having a good reputation, has
the unique advantage of being half an hour from home?
"Thank you so much, we already have a bed at the Curie
and have been referred to an oncologist." "No, no, take
my card. I really do know a lot of people, your son will get
better care. You know, when you don't have any connections..." Now he's seriously bothering me. I know I should
thank him humbly, with a quavering voice and moist eyes,
for the priceless favor he's doing us. And, while I'm at it,

I should admire him for his exceptional social standing as one who rubs shoulders with the best. And then let him play the false modesty card—oh, it's nothing, really, it's only natural. But, well, I don't have the strength for that this morning. I find these little courtesies so draining. I take the card he's proffering and manage a forced thank-you, to get him to leave me in peace. My mother, who has come to sit back down and witnessed the end of the scene, apologizes. She was making a phone call on the café terrace and it was when he overheard her conversation that this man gave himself permission to intervene. We're all a little shaken by his intrusion. Even so, I'm subjected to a few reprimands from my parents for being insufficiently grateful. So I have to get up and go ask the man to forgive my bad manners, justifying them—because, apparently, this wasn't clear enough—with the context of my circumstances. A grotesque situation that stirs further feelings of rebellion in me and teaches me an instant lesson: when it comes to my son's illness, I won't let anyone outside the team caring for him tell me what to do. So they can all come along with their advice, their opinions, their convictions, and their interpersonal skills, driven by kindness, a sense of doing the right thing, or their good conscience, sometimes bolstered by a power complex and suspect motives. The bleeding hearts and the manipulators, the over-emotional and the proud, and, in rather greater numbers, those who are a bit of both. Fate has mapped out my route from Necker to the Curie. I won't listen to another instruction, won't lend an ear to another opinion. The Institute will be my only religion, my creed, my chapel, my church. Indisputably. I have neither the time nor the energy to look elsewhere. My own little scheme for economizing on despair. It hunts down any doubts and drives them out of me. It makes choices for me and leaves me free to act. Free also to crush anything that gets in the way.

The morning vanishes I'm not sure where or doing what. The next place I remember being is on the street level of the Institute in the early afternoon, having waited more than an hour for the ambulance bringing you from Necker. The waiting is unendurable. Filled with absurd paradox. For nearly eighteen hours everyone has been telling us this is a real emergency, but everything seems to be in suspended animation. This contradiction triggers anxiety that evolves into an obsession: your chemotherapy needs to start right now. These words, endlessly repeated like a mantra, keep my mind trussed up in their web, stifling it. It's like a cramp, and I notice its spasms, spaced out at first but progressively concertinaing into continuous convulsions. This cramping remains silent, for want of anyone to talk to, and clenches to the limits of endurance. Soon the stretcher-bearers, nurses, and doctors will suffer the consequences. The trussing will give way, freeing my tensions in uncontrollable repetitions of my litany. But for now everything is held together in the hope of you.

GENESIS

The ambulance finally arrives at about two o'clock.
Your father steps out of it, shattered after a short night
and a long morning. We hug. Then you appear, lying on
a stretcher. Rings around your eyes, your skin pale, your
expression serious. I don't want to think the illness has
changed you already. Besides, everything is brushed away
when I take you in my arms and you smile. I recognize you,
my happy, sunny, living boy. Still, I can't help noticing your
neck: where there was a small protuberance yesterday evening there's now a ball the size of a mandarin. It makes it
difficult for you to open your mouth and alters the way you
speak. My eyes want to avoid it but are drawn to it. Your
chemotherapy needs to start right now. The truss tightens
again, garroting me, suffocating me. Shall we go?

*The pediatric oncology department is on the sixth floor
of the Curie Institute, coming from the entrance on the rue
Louis-Thuillier. To get there you have to take one of the three
elevators whose doors open and close constantly onto the entrance hall. There are two call buttons for them, one featuring
an arrow pointing up, the other an arrow pointing down, depending on whether you want to go to the upper floors or the
basement. If the place is busy, once you've identified your vertical destination, you first need to make a horizontal choice
between the three doors to secure a good spot by the one about*

to open and avoid being rejected by an overfull cabin. Because, for reasons no one seems to understand, these contraptions are particularly slow and apparently capricious. Which means that every missed elevator comes at a price of endless further minutes waiting, thereby increasing the likelihood of meeting figures in pajamas, scrawny incarnations of unbearable physical and psychological decline. Try as they might, on this first day Lise and Olivier identify no logic governing the opening of one door rather than another, and, although they anticipate the likely itinerary of the three elevators by using the numbers signaled above each door, they miss their entry twice. The child grows impatient, whines, seeing this as another nasty trick of fate. It doesn't take long for an anxious mind to interpret this frustrated waiting as some magical curse. The parents meanwhile may also see some distant mythological echoes, some metaphor for an intractable destiny in this crossroads with its random exits visited by dispossessed ghosts. But they don't let a hint of it show. And that's because, although they may be incompetent in elevator systems, they have—in less than forty-eight hours—acquired robust experience of managing anxiety. A game is introduced there and then, one intended to brighten every visit to the Institute for a long time to come. It is based on an inescapable fact: there are three of them, just as there are three of these wretched doors. Each of them can therefore choose a door, then the winner, basking in the pleasure of victory, can invite the other two into his or her cabin, even if that means a bit of elbowing. The competition makes *the waiting manageable and the complicity thwarts their fear. A win-win situation, in fact.*

The trials don't end there. For those who successfully complete this first round, the actual ascent constitutes a second ordeal. Reaching pediatrics, at the very top of the building, means passing all the other floors from bottom to top. On every landing the doors open into a different department, which means that, thanks to the succession of emaciated bodies entering and leaving the elevator, the child can observe at leisure the monstrous metamorphoses of his illness. Strange creatures sidle in among the medical staff, administrators, technicians, and visitors, all of them different and yet instantly distinguishable from the healthy. As if the single trunk of cancer had sprouted a multiplicity of suckers, displaying the infinite variety of its forms in torturous stems, shriveled leaves and withered fruits. On the second floor an old man enters the elevator. He is dried out as sunbaked land. His features are angular, his complexion sallow, his whole face lined with deep creases. He is wearing gray tracksuit pants, a parka in a glum shade of green, and thick woolen socks inside tired old slippers that he drags listlessly over the floor. In fact, he skates more than walks, leaning heavily on the drip pole on which his chemotherapy medication hangs. This haughty metallic pole, raised on casters and with its pouches of liquid connected to the patient through a network of tubes, appears to pull him along rather than him pushing it, preceding each of his hesitant steps like someone dragging a recalcitrant dog on a leash. An acrid smell of tobacco accompanies this strange harnessed pair. The man must have been for a smoke in the gardens and is returning to his room. Lise and Olivier both think that, until the bitter end, addiction gets the better of prudence, even of resentment. On the third floor, the old man leaves and no one enters. It's easier to breathe. On the fourth floor they're joined by a woman. She must be in her early forties, if that. Framed by a blue scarf knotted at the back of her head, her face echoes the diaphanous complexion of Vermeer's girl with a pearl earring. She looks kind. Above all she looks well. At least that's what they're free to believe until the next stop, because when she gets out on the fifth floor, offering a view of her back to those left in the elevator, everyone can see that the scarf is holding back no hair at all. The smooth nape of her neck below the knotted fabric betrays the illness. She is replaced by a young man. Twenty-something, wearing jeans, sneakers, and a white T-shirt with the words "shit happens" on it in black letters. The right sleeve reveals a puny arm while the left hangs empty, folded back on itself. This absence, yet again, traces the contours of an unequal battle. Does the child spend this whole upward journey wondering will he too soon belong to this outlandish species with its motley assemblages? Will he push plastic and metal extensions of himself to one side while superfluous excrescences are amputated from the other, will he dwindle and shrivel, losing his hair and the color in his cheeks along with his strength? That, at least, is what his parents are thinking. And the thought of it ties their stomachs in knots. So, to keep their heads above water, they deliberately concentrate their thoughts on the red numbers flitting over the doors with each passing floor. And sigh with relief when a "6" appears at last and the doors move aside. The young man does not get out, though. Already too old for pediatrics. He lives on the fifth floor, and, probably wanting to go down to the lobby, he took the first elevator that came along, deeming a detour via the sixth floor better than the endless waiting for a cabin on its way down. Sometimes a goal can be achieved only at the cost of bizarre digressions. The child and his parents have to edge past the man to get out. Lise stifles a shudder as she brushes against his shoulder and what remains of his left arm. Never mind. They're here.

The sixth-floor landing offers the newcomer one final decision. It is a T-shaped hallway with the horizontal bar leading on either side to double doors that open onto two distinct networks of further corridors and rooms. A few hours later Lise and Olivier will discover the precise purpose of the two sides and how different—and significant—it is to be treated in one rather than the other. For now, they don't know where to go and hover briefly in front of the wall of photographs facing the elevators. Pictures of bald, bloated, one-eyed, and maimed children in the arms of nurses, Santa Clauses and clowns. All of them happy and smiling. There's definitely something tragic, almost obscene, about the juxtaposition of these two incompatible worlds: suffering and happiness, sickness and childhood. At this early stage, the mother finds the spectacle unbearable. The red of the clowns' cheeks and noses and of the

Santa Claus outfits catches at her heart even more than the scars and the absent hair and limbs.

And, with all this going on, they still have to decide whether to go right or left. A nurse, intercepted as she hurries from one duty to another, points them toward the left-hand corridor where the admissions desk is. They made it, they're here. From this point they're taken under the wing of an experienced administrative, technical, medical, and paramedical team. Secretaries, cleaners, teachers, nurses, doctors, social workers, psychologists, psychiatrists—it turns out a whole little community is waiting to welcome them, question them, inform them, guide them, and direct them. On arrival they don't yet grasp that they are stepping into a world apart, an almost autonomous microcosm with its own operating system, one whose ways and customs they will soon adopt without even realizing it. At the very most they're aware of a fluid sort of authority in its workings, it's not unlike meeting a strong personality. This gives them a sense of relief, and they graciously abdicate their decision-making powers to enter into the programmatic logic of medical protocol. Here, in the Curie Institute's pediatric oncology department, their son's fate will play out in their presence, but independently of them.

Your room is lovely. It smells clean and new and is decorated in harmonious colors, and, best of all, the huge picture window on the south side has peerless views over the Panthéon. I'm amazed to find myself noticing these details, ashamed that I like the superfluous luxury of them, their bourgeois comforts. It wouldn't take much for me to say I was happy to be here. We're going to be okay. I feel frivolous, heartless, stupid, and repulsive to be thinking these things when you could be dead in a few days. I hate myself. At the same time, I imagine this is probably a form of self-defense. Come to think of it, I believe I may be able to help you, to sustain you with these inappropriate, insensitive observations. Perhaps it simply means we can still find pleasure in permitted areas. So I draw your attention to the place, pointing out all the positives, as if we were experts sent by some tourist publication. Television, telephone, view, cleanliness, room service, position, it's at least a four-star, we conclude. I don't hate myself now; I'm playing with you. You've rediscovered your childish curiosity. More than anything else, you're stunned by the Panthéon. You're familiar with its characteristic dome, of course, but from here, a few hundred meters away and filling half our visual field, it looks as if it's been erected for you alone, an arrogant immutable emblem of resistance. You ask me about its history. To great men, recognized by a grateful nation. On this first day of battle, I'm sure you draw strength from this. You too are already a great man, my boy.

Your grandparents have joined us and, *volens nolens*, contribute to our enthusiastic appraisal of the room. I can see the pain and fear in their eyes. You find a card game on the windowsill. Superior four-star room. It's an unusual deck, featuring distinctive round cards and requiring memory and visual concentration. It consists in recognizing the common element among the dozens of illustrations featured on the cards that all the players turn over at the same time. You play with your grandfather and you're thrilled to win every hand. Your father, grandmother, and I savor your boisterous pleasure and are impressed by your quick wits. Your brain's working fine. I feel as if I'm watching your super-quick neuronal connections in real time, a blossoming of flashing lights culminating in the final explosion of your triumphant laugh. I can't seem to understand that the machine of your body, with all the perfection and promise of childhood, now finds itself invaded by a degenerative inanity that is gradually necrotizing it. I can't reconcile the insolent life force of your youth with this old-man sickness produced by wear and tear, by cellular damage, and yet that *is* what they say you have. I find the incoherence of it outrageous, but it still leaves me with a profound sense of your invincibility.

We stay in the room for an uncharted length of time, and then someone comes for us. It's time for our first meeting with the oncologist. We leave your grandparents in the room and the three of us head for the consulting room at the other end of the corridor. Dr. O sees us there. Late forties, quite tall, black hair, kind of friendly-looking. I stare right at him. So your life will depend on this man. On his interpretations, his decisions, his experience. I need to respect him enough to put my trust in him alone. I hope he'll help me with that. He sits at his desk and turns his chair to the side. We seat ourselves facing him on three chairs placed next to each other along the side wall, with you in the middle. This layout maps out a first feeling of familiarity. And yet I get the sense that his moves and this arrangement, even down to the deliberately relaxed mood, fulfill carefully studied protocol requirements. This is confirmed when two nurses come and sit on either side of our group, one beside your father, the other beside me. Are they here to lessen the initial blow? To catch us if we collapse? To stall a potential scene? Minders of mind and body. In any event, the dice are loaded. Because these precautions are probably intended for the first announcement. The one when, after all the medical examinations, the parents are seen for the first time and told the results. The one when, with well-chosen words and appropriate facial expressions, ensuring the correct balance is maintained between empathy and restraint, good people are told that their child has a potentially fatal illness. The one when, without batting too much of an eyelid, some hope must be offered even while the tragedy is revealed. Whereas we have in fact been denied precisely this inaugural framework. The announcement has already been made: truncated, inappropriate, and shockingly badly delivered. And this whole setup comes

47

too late. All we had were a few words on the phone, then silence and the unendurable waiting at Necker. No thoughtful welcome, no speechified warnings, no eye contact, no outstretched hand. Alone on the threshold. So what's the point of all this ceremony now? Why repeat in more decorous terms today what we were dealt so unceremoniously yesterday? It's almost comic. But what does it matter in the end, given that the unbearable has already been said and the harm done? They can go ahead and add whatever they like. I've been through the worst.

How naive I am. I haven't yet grasped that the worst is yet to come. Dr. O crosses his legs and leans in. The hem of his pants lifts to reveal, on his left sock, Tex Avery's Road Runner and the coyote. This has the same effect on me as the Santa Clauses at the entrance to the department. Incongruous and out of place. That's a minus. I don't want a playmate for my son. I have glimpses of limited emotional scope, of nostalgia for childhood and professional compensation. A flaw. I try to drive away the idea, along with any attendant reflections on the secret motives that might lead someone to choose a career in which you see one child in five succumb. Fundamental altruism, a masochist tendency to self-abnegation, compensating for a personal tragedy, a need for total power, even a slight element of sadism? Nevertheless, I feel a wave of sympathy for Dr. O. I wouldn't like to be in his shoes right now. To look us in the eye—we the parents of three young children, worthy adults

and honest citizens, full of moral integrity and promise—
and have to tell us something so appalling. For a moment
I almost pity him. I understand how incredibly difficult it
must be to find the right tone of voice, choose the right
words, gauge the right degree of distance. It must be exhausting. In fact, it nearly excuses the gaffe with the socks.
Or at least explains it. I want to help him, to tell him not
to go to the trouble, we already know. And to reassure him
too. We'll behave ourselves. We'll maintain our dignity
and do exactly what's required of us. Then my brain goes
over everything again. Actually, there's no need to worry
about him. I don't want to think of the man in front of me
in any other way than the objectivity of his role. He simply
has to be the best oncologist in the world and to save my
son's life. I couldn't care less about anything else. I eye him
again. He half opens his mouth. There's no more need for
thinking now. He's going to speak.

"Hello, I'm Doctor O. I'm going to be looking after
you. So, tell me, what's your name?" Not a bad start. It
feels direct and reassuring. But still the tension mounts.
Everything seems to freeze in the brief ensuing pause. As
if the future depends on the answer to this everyday question. You look at the doctor for a moment and then with
unwavering eyes but a shaky voice, you say very quietly:
"Solal." Oh, it's such a strong, beautiful name. So strong
and beautiful that it's barely been whispered into the room
before it smooths and settles the metallic tension in the air.

Long before you were born, Solal, I had a vision of you inspired by Albert Cohen's *Belle du Seigneur*: I saw you as a luminous young man in the midday sun, dismounting a horse and stepping, strange and princely, through hazels and dog roses, almost victorious already. Yes Solal, Solal of all Solals, I pictured you in the diffuse brilliance of sunlight, a great lord in tall boots, noble and stately, dancing gracefully among the animals and spring flowers. Solal again, So-la-l, from your first few hours on earth I let your cluster of notes resonate, composing a tender lullaby to see you through the night. "So, so, so, so much sunshine over la, la, la, land and sea. So, so, so, my little Solal, I la, la, la, love you so, so, so." And it wasn't until years after knowing its sounds and letters that I discovered the meaning of this name I'd chosen for you—you, Solal, the first child with a surname that means "blessed by the gods": I'd unwittingly given you a name anchored in your Hebrew legacy, marking out your primary position among your siblings. Solal, "the pathfinder," a triumphant pioneer, a sunny melodious incipit. Definitely too strong and beautiful for this cramped consulting room. How can this grim, sterile impersonal setting accommodate the joyful majesty of your two syllables? It knows nothing of the laughter of exceptional youth. Any more than it does of the tangled motionless forest, of the clearing by the riverbanks, the iridescent shimmer on the water, the echoing sounds lulling the soul, or the first conquests and elemental splendors. It even knows nothing of my love. Nothing will be left but age-old fear. Nothing will have happened but this lifeless moment, cloistered in this hospital cubbyhole, stifled in the cloak of heartbreak that is enfolding your existence. Even your answer is eventually lost in the deafening silence.

Dr. O then tries, tentatively, to piece you together. Age, school class, hobbies, friends, illusory fragments, vanishing points before impact. We really do need to get down to it. "Well, Solal, you know why you're here?" His intonation is unusual, almost making me wonder whether this is a question or a statement. Either way, Dr. O provides his own answer. "You're sick, Solal, you have cancer." A left uppercut straight to my stomach. He caught me off guard. I feel my chest collapse and my body recoil. It knocks the breath out of me. For twenty-four hours now I've been telling you there's something wrong with your blood, deliberately avoiding the word "cancer." Because, being so widespread, the word no longer has a precise meaning. Because, by referring to hundreds of different pathologies and by erasing the differences between them, it now means nothing but a possibly tragic outcome. Because, in more concrete terms, for the last ten years your grandfather has been battling a cancer that's now getting the better of him and I would never want you to confuse the fight you're about to have with this promise of defeat. "Cancer." How could he, without even considering what we've already told you, start with that? The protocol most likely insists on facts and candor. I understand that. But then I'd have preferred him to be precise and to use the exact name of your illness: lymphoma. Lymphoma, a paradoxically delicate and melodious word. It would have made you think of lynxes, nymphs, foam, frothy legendary words to fuel daydreams. Unless, limp foe that it is, it gave you a poetic means to detect the enemy's fleeting, cowardly figure. But cancer, no. You too have taken it right in the guts. I felt you cave in next to me. You slumped in an instant, like a puppet whose strings have been cut. Your head has dropped onto your chest. Your fingers are twisted together, creating a misshapen structure. You're now terribly small, serious, and still. I hug you to me. This pain that's being dealt to you hurts me so much. I don't know what you're told next. I don't even know whether you and Dr. O say anything else. He probably tells you about the treatment. Whatever it is, it's brief. And yes, I can see you leaving the room moments later and going back to your grandparents in your room. Your father and I have to stay here. The time has come for the truth.

Lise doesn't speak. She has nothing to say. This man's every word is like a punch to her stomach. She feels the physical violence of them. In fact she has folded in two, arms crossed, shoulders hunched, as if to protect herself. In this position, she would need to extend her neck and raise her head to look at the doctor. But she would rather keep her head down while he beats her up. She is stunned and hardly moves. A little shiver just runs through her with each new piece of information. Not that she's assimilating what she's being told. She definitely heard, at the start, that they were dealing with a non-Hodgkin lymphoma and, although she didn't really grasp what this meant, she understood that this negative definition was not in their favor. She also quickly realized that every sentence was freighted with its own share of suffering and risks. But right now, she doesn't understand any of it. The sentences accumulate, piling up like so many impersonal rulings on the desk of a meticulous judge. In the end the very meaning of words is beyond her. On the other hand, her body has picked up on the rhythm of this bout. It knows that the punches stop every time the voice drops, then, after a brief respite, they start again when the voice does, growing increasingly fierce as the time periods grow longer. And so it prepares to endure these successive attacks and simply wait until they stop.

Olivier meanwhile hasn't faltered. He has stayed upright on his chair, sitting tall on his ischium bones, his hands crossed on his thighs and his chest slightly inclined toward the doctor. He listens attentively and asks countless questions, dozens of them, concrete, targeted, relevant questions. It's as if no emotion whatsoever hampers his thoughts. His interventions are so clear and pertinent that he even seems to have developed a sort of intellectual hyperacuity. Lise is amazed by this ability, almost begrudges it for operating so well precisely when she is foundering disastrously, although she is also grateful that she can rely on her husband's efficacious memory. The couple will not discuss this scene and their remarkably contradictory reactions until years later. Olivier will then admit to Lise that, at the time of the conversation, he had no awareness of the reality of the subjects, having not yet assimilated the fact that his son had cancer. He will therefore acknowledge that his attention to detail was all the more acute because he had no sense of what was at stake.

Neither of the parents, then, truly partakes in the discussion. But what can they really glean from it anyway? Months, years of uncertainty. Their child's body endlessly attacked with the most aggressive forms of chemotherapy to fight the most aggressive of cancers. No hair left, no defenses left, no more food, no more home, no more school, no more childhood. Tubes in his chest to introduce treatments and nourishment, giant needles in his back to test his cells and inject other treatments, weeks on end of hospitalization to receive chemotherapy, and immediately after that further weeks to treat its destructive side effects and get the body back in shape, and these themselves immediately followed by yet more weeks of chemotherapy. A vicious circle of care and devastation, with no end in sight. Because here's the paradox: the very treatment that is to heal this child must also partially—but as a matter of priority—strike him down. Still, the parents must remain alert if, behind these evocations of the galloping enemy and the massive weapons used to tackle it, they are to have glimpses of a possible recovery. But right now their minds have fled the scene.

When Lise leaves the room she does at least see why the two nurses are here. Their job is to gather up what strength this conversation has left her. And it is in fact at this point, aided and abetted by their thoughtful gestures and empathetic looks, that the truss that has been torturing her insides finally releases its grip. Coldly and mechanically, her anxiety unravels. The sudden expansion resolves itself into an uninterrupted flow of muttered words: "His chemo needs to start right now. Why didn't they start it yesterday? What are they waiting for to inject the stuff into him? Why waste time talking? What's happened to all that urgency?" The nurses explain, again. Standing there in the corridor, they go back over some of what has been said, but with such clear, supple, deft words that the mother finally manages to hear them. Since yesterday Solal has been on a constant cortisone drip to slow the progress of the cancer cells. Cortisone is one of the substances used in the chemotherapy protocol. A form of treatment has therefore started. But not every aspect of the treatment can be delivered by drip. His veins wouldn't take it. Which is why a central catheter needs to be set up into a large vein near his heart. It is installed during surgery, under general anesthetic. This will happen tomorrow. The anesthetist is waiting for them now for a preparatory consultation in the basement.

3

You're sitting on a blue plastic chair. You're staring at a point on the floor. Lined up next to you are more plastic chairs, connected by small metal hooks. Other people sit waiting on these chairs, and they too are frozen in some form of despair, at their saddest. I know they are there but don't see them. They're adults, most of them elderly. You're the only child in this basement room in the Institute. Here, more than ever, I appreciate the scandalous incongruity of this cancerous degeneration in your young body. Every morsel of space in the room distorts, folds, and converges on you. Or rather the absence of you. A solemn figure, an expressionless face, empty eyes. You're more than motionless. You're a gaping black hole.

You turned ten three weeks ago. But that was before. When you still laughed, when you were gorgeous and radiant. When you still cried over innocent injuries and crises. When you could still be a child, just a child. That was another life, irretrievably vandalized two hours ago.

"You must feel like a building fell on top of you."

A brief pause. You look up. I must keep going.

"What do you think it's made of, then, this building?"

"It's made of lead." There. You spoke, you're here, you're back. Now we can start to fight.

"You're not going to carry this building on your own, you know. There'll be a bunch of people to help you. Mommy and Daddy, your brother and sister, family, friends, school, doctors, and all the medical staff. And plus everything you like and will still be able to do. That's a lot of arms to hold up the building and lighten your load. So, of course at the beginning it's you this is happening to. You're the one who has to deal with the illness, and you'll probably be left with something to carry, but it won't be a lead building, a little cabin lost in the woods at the very most. Maybe just a straw house that you could blow away with one puff."

"Like in 'The Three Little Pigs'?"

"Like in 'The Three Little Pigs.'" First victory. Your imagination's working again. It's slow and apathetic to start. A question where once—only two hours ago—there would have been a gush. A memory, rather than an invention. Then the cogs gradually set in motion and, although you still look serious, you start contentedly listing a wacky collection of light, airy materials to substitute for the lead. Cardboard, sponge, foam, paper, polystyrene, net curtains, parachute silk, feathers. There we go.

You soon stop, though. Too soon. Go back to the point on the floor. The solemn figure, the expressionless eyes, the empty face. And your fingers that you keep wringing compulsively. That's it. You've gone again, I lost you again. A second absence, prefiguring so many others. I need to go back to the grindstone. I already know I'll have to go back to it a hundred times, a thousand times.

"And then one day there'll be nothing left to carry, not even the dumbest little shack. Not even its shadow. Nothing, do you hear that, nothing at all. You will have won."

I don't have time to see your reaction, the nurse is calling us, it's our turn.

The anesthetist examines you, listens to your chest and weighs you. He explains, in detail, how the port-a-cath will be installed. A small appliance is implanted under the skin and connected to a catheter that runs into the vena cava. Treatments can then be injected into it with a Huber needle. You'll have two scars, one tiny one below your collarbone, and the other slightly larger but hidden under your armpit. Right now, I don't really take in what this is about. It all goes too quickly. Before understanding the technical workings of the equipment, I'd first like to understand its name. I can't get beyond thinking of "Cath" as a person's name and don't realize it's an abbreviation of "catheter." Then there's the expression "implant chamber" that the doctor keeps bandying about. The combination of the two terms produces nothing coherent. I have images of secret dark alcoves where this foreign object will make its intrusion into my child's body. I need to be shown one of these chambers, so that I can get a handle on the shape of it, appreciate the size of it, and feel the substance of it. Instead of this, the anesthetist hands me a document several pages long, describing the procedure and stating the possible complications. And, as is now required for every surgical procedure, however minor, I have to take responsibility for the risk. There's a diagram on the first page: two thin parallel lines inside two wider lines leading into an ovoid shape. They're going to touch your heart. Stop. I refuse to go any further. I don't want to know any more. What *is* the point of making us read these forms and sign these disclaimers? I don't understand any of it, anyway. The lines blur before my eyes; the words don't make sense. My brain is not available. It isn't a tool for analyzing and processing. It's a machine that takes in facts, then gives instructions or the most appropriate response to each stimulus. A mechanism with no soul. Besides, what does the meaning of words matter? They can inventory all the risks and list the hemorrhages, infections, pneumothoraxes, occlusions, cardiac disturbances, and other side effects as much as they like, do I really have the option to refuse? These are just potential dangers, extremely rare negligible statistics. But without the port-a-cath, without the treatments, without my accepting the risks, your death is guaranteed. One hundred percent. And imminent too. So of course I sign right away, without reading through, without taking advantage of the thinking time I'm offered. What good would it do to add fear to the horror, when this is just about giving the medical staff legal protection. The real question is binary: 0 you die, 1 you live. I choose 1, and I don't really care what happens between the two. The procedure is scheduled for early afternoon tomorrow. We're getting somewhere.

When we get back to your room there's a nasty surprise waiting for us. We have to move out. We didn't know it but we were in transit, in the outpatient department. This isn't where you'll be having your treatments. They need a more permanent setup. So we have to move over to the other side, to inpatients. It's a painful process. Not that it's materially complicated to cross that frontier. We brought nothing with us. We're traveling light. But at the time of the first traumas, this room's comforts stood in for familiarity. Coping with another new space is a pointless call on my energy. I'll have to start from scratch finding exceptional qualities, grounds for delight, and reasons to hope in the very place that's assaulting us. This apparently trifling effort establishes the paradigm for the next few months, a laborious struggle to spare you the instabilities of reality. Although I don't realize it, the spiral shaft of exhaustion is starting its slow drilling process, boring into me progressively with each of my restorative words and gestures. And yet there's nothing else to say or do. So here we are retracing our steps. Back to the landing with the elevators, back to square one, to this place of uncertainty and waiting where your identity as a sick person is still searching for definition, a place suspended between fear and impatience. We've explored the left-hand wing of this floor and we've been down to the basement; now it's time to go through the double doors on the right to reach our destination at last.

At first there's nothing, no one. A bench seat, a feebly illuminated aquarium, a few magazines. Then a drip comes over, green and white pouches hanging from its hooks. I search for some trace of life at the end of the tubes. I can barely make it out behind the tangle of steel and plastic. It's a little girl, a baby, about eighteen months old. She's pushing the wheeled contraption, almost running, while also using it for support. She's turned this scaffold into a baby walker. She's laughing. Her skull is hairless and cut across, ear to ear, by a huge scar. Her left eyelid is closed and abnormally concave. Covering a void. Eyeless. Shrieks ring out. They make us jump, then scoot right past us along with two figures on the floor. Four wheels, a red seat, two sets of pedals, and two children, sitting one behind the other, nearly knock us over and careen across the corridor, hurtling toward outpatients, execute a screeching U-turn at the end of the corridor, almost knock us over again on the way back, and end their breakneck trip alongside the wall facing us, among various other tricycles and karts. We chicane around the obstacle to set off along another corridor at a right angle. To our right a table-soccer table, on our left a piano. Between the two an uninterrupted coming and going of white uniforms and unfamiliar creatures. But emphatically children. Many of them are bald. Some are missing an eye, an arm, or a leg. Most of them drag drips, with some difficulty. The casters catch in electric cables, get stuck in doorways, or seize for no reason. Progress is often tentative. One little boy stops not far from us. He snatches a cardboard bowl, a sort of gray bean into which he vomits in a succession of retches. He looks as if he's going to collapse. A nurse hurries over to help him, addressing us with an embarrassed smile. She takes the bean with one hand and with the other helps the child, who now leans all his weight on the drip. This peculiar crew heads off again, turns first to the right, then to the left, walking away and disappearing into a part of the department we don't yet know. A high-pitched sound suddenly starts up, and persists, continuous and penetrating. It's an A, high A. I instinctively turn to the piano. No one. The sound doesn't fade, though. It's almost as if it's coming closer and intensifying. I find its persistence even more grueling than the strident pitch. I want it to end, this instant. It's really close now, almost menacing. I turn around, panicking. Facing me is the baby we saw at the entrance. The scar, the missing eye, the drip and its tubes clustered into a large gray box that's blinking in time to the sound. So that's where it's coming from. A young woman runs over, kisses the child, says a few words to her in a language I don't understand, presses on the box, walks around us, kneels at our feet, picks up an electric lead, and plugs it into a socket in the corridor. The noise stops, instantly. I can breathe.

Where are they? When Lise and Olivier arrive at the inpatient department, nothing matches their expectations. This is because they have hastily—in the space of so few hours—put together an erroneous image of the intended treatment, woven from the embryonic snatches of information at their disposal: the identity of the illness, medical information, and brightly colored images of pediatric oncology. They've been promised an intensive protocol over six months or a year, with virtually continuous hospitalization due to the frequent iterations of total aplasia. Long periods when the child will have no immune defenses because, they have been told, it is his lymphocytes— precisely the cells that should be fighting illness and infection— that have gone crazy. In order for their son to be cured, this much they understand, his entire arsenal of weapons against invasive organisms needs to be destroyed several times over. Creating a risk of septicemia each time. They have therefore been picturing their child in a transparent bubble, isolated from the outside world, protected by a perfectly sealed airlock that nothing can penetrate. A pure, white, silent universe. How can this overpopulated, cacophonous place correspond in any way to this service? Everything about it seems unrestricted and out of control. As with any organized system that has been desta-bilized, the violent effect this illness is having on them has fostered a sort of totalitarian xenophobia in them. They long for boundaries, demarcations, and no-go zones. They aspire to a secure sanctuary, to thoroughly hygienic orderliness. They want nothing more than to be left alone with their pain. Truth be told, they might manage to adapt to the justifiable sound of the machines and the toing and froing of medical staff; they might possibly even tolerate the presence of other sick children. But what are all the rest of them doing here, all these people who have nothing to do with cancer? By what right do they come in here, bringing in the whole miasma of the outside world? Seasonal viruses and microbes exhaled on fetid breath, bacteria and parasites deposited with every gesture, garbage, filth, excretions, sidewalk sediment brought in on their shoes, sickening smells of tobacco, sweat, or perfume fouling the air, shocking intrusions all of them, and potential bearers of death. And now, feeling threatened, their souls become despotic, tracking down dirt and already identifying these scapegoats. They don't spare themselves from this tyranny, though. They are well aware that they are by nature part of this exogenous world from which their child must be protected. And it is not the least of the horrors besetting them that they loathe them-selves for this: doubting the harmlessness of a tender gesture, despising the very demonstrations of their love. The mother has already mourned this passing. Confronted with despotic sterilization, she has immediately accepted the sacrifice. And

GENESIS

she claims that, for the sake of this sterility, when the time comes, she will be prepared to forbid herself from taking her child in her arms, kissing his hands, or his face, even talking to him. Prepared to stay behind the window for months to help him from afar, having no negative impact, prepared to cherish him remotely, transparently.

But it turns out that's not where they're at. A nurse comes to greet them. She is young and pretty, and her name is Julie. She bends toward Solal with a smile. She is to be his principal caregiver in the first few days of his treatment. She offers to take him to his room. The parents and their child follow her, they pass the piano, walk three yards to the right and one to the left, then come to a stop—already—by an open door at the very beginning of a long corridor. They enter a largish room furnished with one bed, on which a little girl is playing, a screen, and a second, empty bed. Julie explains in veiled terms that newcomers are usually given single rooms, but because Solal's case is urgent they've had to make this arrangement. At the time neither Olivier nor Lise appreciates what this apparently harmless concession implies in extra stress. For now they're glad to have arrived. As with the previous room, Lise makes an effort to list its plus points, its promise of comforting moments to come. So the room is huge thanks to the fact it's shared, it's practical for being at the front end of the corridor, fun because it's near the piano and the table-soccer table, and alive because it's noisy. But her heart isn't in it and this inventory doesn't ring true. Succumbing to exhaustion, Lise lies

65

down on the empty bed without thinking. She's so tired she's forgotten the elementary rules of hygiene, unless, floundering in her heartbreak, she's tempted literally to take her son's place by doing this. The nurse gently brings her to her senses, then calls for two members of staff to change the sheets and remake the bed. Embarrassed, the mother apologizes profusely and feels utterly helpless. She can't think what to say. A tide of questions sweeps over her and the feeling of urgency—and its concomitant anxiety—resurfaces.

In this context, Dr. O's arrival comes at first as a relief. This is, however, short-lived. He lays the child down on the bed and examines him. Solal finds it difficult to open his mouth, and harder still to talk. It hurts. His parents look away. Now that their son is in the hospital they no longer want to witness the thing's monstrous distortions for themselves. They will never know what the affected tonsil has become on this second day. They won't know if it now reaches beyond the middle of his throat, pushing the uvula aside and coming to join its twin. Neither will they know whether the black threads have totally covered it, whether there is any visible pink flesh left, whether necrosis has won the battle. They will never know, and they come to terms with this. The clinical examination doesn't give rise to any comments. Dr. O simply reminds them of the procedure for tomorrow's intervention and what will come next. Once again, the mother understands nothing. She can't even formulate the questions that, moments ago, badgered at her mind. Strangely, they *seem to escape her now, like shapes half-identified through a fog so that when they vanish there is no certainty they were there at all. And then there's that noise that's stopping her thinking. A nasal clicking against a background of intermingled voices. The regular beat of it soon becomes maddening, fragmenting the doctor's words like hiccups, chopping them into chaotic syllables. It fills every inch of space and precludes any concentration. Unable to understand him, Lise still makes an effort to look at the doctor, for fear of offending him. But her eyes are constantly drawn elsewhere, hoping to identify the source of the noise. Which is quickly done: the little girl on the neighboring bed behind the screen is playing a video game, while cartoons play on loop on the TV hanging from the wall between the two beds. There's nothing to say. Lise fastens her eyes on the doctor's mouth again. She doesn't understand a thing, but at least plays the part. Which is how she is ready, once the doctor falls silent, to reprise her litany about urgency. Why wait till tomorrow to install the port-a-cath? Why not start the protocol straightaway? What's the point of leaving the cancerous cells to develop like this? These questions, which have now become familiar, are probably in some way reassuring for the mother. Not so much in terms of the answers they solicit—answers that have been given many times over since the day before—but simply by their repetition. A consoling and sedative lament. The oncologist, a seasoned expert, most likely understands the role they play, because he consents to repeat the same answers, unruffled.*

Then he leaves, setting another appointment with the parents
for after the intervention.

I can't take any more. Of the pandemonium, the bustle, the
confusion, the aggressive sounds, and the visions of horror
in this freak show. I so can't take any more that I can't even
feel it. I don't feel much at all, in fact, apart from a distinct
difficulty breathing. After the oncologist's visit I leave the
room and sit on a small, light-colored wooden bench in the
corridor. It faces the long row of closed doors behind which
other sick children wage their battles. I stare at a point off
in the distance. I'm reduced to nothing. And sit frozen to
the spot, absent. My mother comes over gently, puts a hand
on my arm, and says, "I think it's time you went home."
Home, she's right, I'd forgotten.

Lise doesn't remember the journey home that evening. And
yet it must have felt strange being back outside the hospital.
Leaving behind the closed world of the department. And,
along with the patients and their caregivers, leaving behind
the smells of vomit and sanitization. Feeling the city's chill
air, meeting unscathed people and healthy children, hearing
conversations, gossip, and laughter. Perhaps feeling surprise

that the world keeps going, in spite of everything. Cars keep on moving, shops keep on selling, gripers keep on griping. Past the initial surprise, this probably afforded her a form of relief. Not everything foundered when she was shipwrecked. And sunk though she may be, she herself is a part of this activity. She can still walk in the street, avoid danger, make out people's faces, smile at acquaintances, stand tall and proud. In fact, there's nothing to differentiate her from other Parisians. No one knows. Not the woman in the bakery on the corner, nor the passerby clamped to his cell phone, nor the neighbor who gives her a quick wave. There is no visible sign of her ordeal. No scarlet letter stitched to her chest. The wound is secret. Her suffering travels incognito. Lise may not remember the trip home, then, but she does know that it was decisive. In fact, it is most likely on this trip, confronted with this world in which she does and yet does not belong, that she recovers her strength. Because the École Normale still stands on the rue d'Ulm, the elementary school on the rue de l'Arbalète, the grocery store on the rue Claude-Bernard, the bookshop on rue Édouard-Quénu, and the gate to their house on rue P. Because everything has been shaken up but nothing has changed. All her ardor is probably shut away in the little nugget of misery and pain trapped at the Institute. Being the mother of a child with cancer most likely entails forced modifications to her identity. But here she still is, in the middle of the city, an anonymous individual. And she can tell that this anonymity will afford her freedom.

When she arrives home, Lise is suffused with a different type of energy. She is reunited with Nils and Anna, who throw themselves at her. They hug her briefly, then dance around her, giving a giddying rundown of the day's events. Like a pair of puppies yapping eagerly to greet her. They have a lovely smell of school, canteens, recess. They too give her an opportunity to breathe the air of the outside world. Most of all they remind her that, as well as being mother to a child with cancer, she is still mother to two healthy children. In their company Lise is a little surprised to realize how comforting she finds routine activities—things usually associated with tiredness. They ensure permanence amid the chaos, and focus her attention as she sways dizzily above the abyss. But it's a permanent struggle, and it's not easy to stay on course. She constantly has to stop herself deviating, and achieves this by stringing together homework, bath time, pajamas, and dinner, avoiding any downtime. Grabbing hold of her thoughts and hauling them back to the here and now. This takes a colossal effort at first. It seems to go against nature, because a constrained mind appears bound to keep trying to escape. But it soon becomes automatic. Over the next few hours, a pendulum motion starts to regulate Lise's mental functions. Every swing toward the Institute spontaneously returns to the house, then sets off again to visit the sick child. And Lise begins to feel that she is the vertical, the calibrated axis of this pendulum. At the same time, she understands that, to ease the movement's abrupt action, she must limit its amplitude. Too much distance creates *tension, and tension produces a painful impact. So when she's at home she must be careful, if not to forbid herself thinking about the Curie, then to keep the two different worlds sufficiently close. Subject to the appropriate gravitational force, the swinging then becomes more harmonious. The succession of polar extremes, the retraced trajectories, and the constant mobility constitute a new form of inertia for her. It presupposes something close to acceptance. Solal's illness and the uncertainties and pain that go along with it are now integral parts of their life. And this means they need to rethink the way their family works around this intruder.*

Lise is not immediately aware of this. It evolves stealthily while she automatically carries out her everyday chores. It is only at the end of the evening, once Anna and Nils are asleep, that the question takes shape. Lise is in the bathtub. For a long time she will wonder what peculiar but necessary initiative urged her to cosset herself like this on this particular evening, warming the room, dimming the lights, ringing her nakedness with a few water lily–shaped floating candles. She feels instantly soothed. And this allows her thoughts and emotions to circulate freely. She doesn't steer her thoughts but settles for observing their ebb and flow, chaotic and rushed at first then gradually slowing and becoming more orderly. From an appropriate distance, she witnesses her successive feelings while her heartbeat settles to a nonchalant rhythm. She is overcome by a strange sense of peace, in spite of everything. Is it exhaustion from the day, the warmth in the bathroom, or some unsuspected resilience? She has no idea. One thing she does know, though, is that this feeling of dissolution eventually fosters an unexpected concentration of will. Something definitely happens. A sort of mental shift, something clicks, and she will say later she as good as heard the sound it made in her head. As if, taking advantage of her abandon, she has activated a switch deep inside her mind. She is suddenly hyper-lucid. In a flash she knows exactly what she must do, what she must say, who she must be, with Solal, with the other children, with Olivier, with her family, her friends, people in general. She studies the crystal-clear facts of her future. She doesn't think she has ever felt so sure of anything. Not simply the feeling that she will win this battle, but an illusory but fundamental conviction of her own essential invincibility. It would make her head spin were it not for the very fact that she feels unshakable. She is exactly where she needs to be. The axis runs through her, keeping her upright, strong and unbending. She won't deviate until her son is saved.

Her resolve forms a basis for courage and provides fertile ground for action. Obstacles diminish of their own accord. Knotty issues untangle. In light of this new assurance, what first struck Lise as hostile now becomes familiar. The Institute isn't far from home. Why can't it be the apartment in the Fifth Arrondissement that they've always dreamed of but never been able to afford? Better still, a second home, an extension of their apartment, where the family can get together in the evenings after school, on weekends, or during holidays.

A hospitable space. As for the bustle, the coming and going, the pandemonium that besieged them when they first arrived there, Lise now recognizes the assets these are. They are life itself. An opportunity to be grasped. And this can start as of tomorrow, Wednesday, children's day because they have a half day at school. Given that it's a turbulent world, Nils and Anna can take part in its commotion, can cycle up and down the corridors, squeal over the table soccer, play piano, laugh out loud as they slalom between the drips. Towing Solal along with them in their exuberance. Together the three of them can go exploring in the playroom that she and Olivier have been told about but have not yet seen. Yes, tomorrow they'll all go to the Curie. As she goes into bed this evening Lise can't wait for it to be morning, when she can take her son in her arms and reconstitute their invincible family unit around him.

4

Wednesday, December 19. Day Three.

Your sister is sitting in the kitchen on the rush-seat chair. She recently turned seven. Nils sits facing her on a pale wooden stool. He is just four. It's morning and the three of us are having breakfast. Your father stayed the night with you. I'm trying to maintain a semblance of routine to reconnect us with life: we chat about our hot chocolate, the spreads on our toast, school, the upcoming holidays. And then Anna mentions you: she wants to see you, she misses you. I suggest that we go this very morning, if they'd like to. The two of them are thrilled with the idea. Joy returns to our household, for a while. But Anna soon looks downhearted again and asks, "What exactly is wrong with Solal? Because," she continues with a hint of exasperation, "all his friends at school keep asking what's wrong with him and all his friends is like the whole school. And I had enough of it." I don't hesitate for a moment, I know exactly what I must tell her. You've been told, it's time your brother and sister knew. I can't let them go on believing you just need your tonsils out. Nor can I let them keep hoping that we'll all be going to Morocco in three days as planned. "He has a type of cancer, it's called lymphoma." For a moment I'm blindingly aware how surreal it is to have a conversation like this with such young children. I need to get down to concrete facts quickly and explain, but I don't have time to add anything that might soften the news. Anna has already asked the only real question: "Is he going to die?" I'm not shocked by it, not surprised by it, not even stressed by it. There, I've tipped into another reality, a world where little girls can ask their mothers whether their brothers are going to die. Is Anna even a little girl still as we have this conversation? The three of us in this kitchen are suddenly projected outside time and relative ages. Of course I try to find words that children will understand, but the truth I'm relaying to them has only one name. It will tolerate no lies or concealment. And so I give the apparently innocuous reply that the oncologist gave us yesterday: "It can be treated." This exemplar of the implicit statement, which says everything without saying anything, feels appropriate. By using these words, am I hoping to deceive myself and deceive my children? Am I secretly hoping to leave it at that? But that wouldn't allow for the pertinence of Anna's questions, or their impertinence, a combination of emotional acuity and intellectual rigor. Perhaps, contrariwise, I'm so sure she'll take this further that I've risked an open-ended reply in the subconscious hope of saying the truth. The ball is in my daughter's court; she gets right onto it. "But what if it doesn't work?" "It can be treated," I say again. My intonation is slightly different this time, firmer, more emphatic. I know that Anna has understood the words in their complexity. I know she's glimpsed the abyss of conditionality opening up beneath that "can be." An abyss in which chance can always come and play its part. Perhaps I think that by reiterating these words I can still haul them back to some unequivocal meaning. "But what if it doesn't work?" Anna asks again. This time I take more drastic action. "There are no ifs." I'm not lying. I'm not talking about the illness now, nor the treatment or the risks. I'm talking about my war, my strategy, and my plan of attack. And there is only one possible outcome in this war. So, from that vantage point, there really are no ifs. But Anna is still here and gracefully tempers my ardor. Her eyes alight with intensity and with a soft smile on her lips she tactfully delivers these irrefutable words: "And if that mockingbird don't sing, and if that looking glass gets broke, and if that billy goat won't pull . . . You see, Mom, there's a lot of ifs."

Anna has said it all. The conversation could stay there, hanging from that melody, but I have to get back to the emergencies of the real world. Time really is of the essence. In an hour we'll be at the Institute. And there will be more than just curiosity, games, and the pleasure of being reunited: your brother and sister will be stepping into the freak show. They'll meet the one-eyed girl with the scar over her scalp. They'll see faltering toddlers, and will walk past maimed teenagers. They'll picture you like these other children someday. And quite rightly. Because we've been warned. In a week's time we won't recognize you. You'll be bald, weak, vomiting, in pain, hospitalized three-quarters of the time, and you'll be treated, fed, and constantly escorted by a tangle of tubes. This regime will last six months to a year, if all goes well. If. So on the doorstep I stop suddenly. I'm struck, again, by a fear of tainting. But this time it's Anna and Nils I want to protect. I don't want the horror of it to contaminate their fresh-eyed gaze, or the pain to impregnate their souls. I wish they didn't even have to know the possibility of it. But I already have no choice about that. The wheels are in motion, the route is mapped out. We've all set off on the journey. We have to take it on, together. I feel I must lay down some ground rules on the subject right away, sort of strategic verbal warnings. Firstly, to differentiate your illness from the one that's taking your grandfather from us. Without saying that it's much worse, of course. And to achieve this, I must outmaneuver the homonymy, dissociate words and things. Four, seven, and ten—that's young to be introduced to doubt. Never mind, we're going to win. Secondly, make you understand that the very thing that attacks your body, changes the way you look, and compromises you physically is the one and only solution to cure you. Every bout of nausea, every mouth ulcer, every sign of weakness, even every pain will be one more step toward victory. We must ignore the evidence yet again. Four, seven, and ten—that's young to understand complexity. Never mind, we're going to win. Finally recognizing the solitary and yet collective nature of the fight. You are at the center of it but Anna and Nils are personally affected too, and will therefore have every right to complain, to scream about how unfair it is, to hate the whole world, including you. Whatever they say, we'll be there to listen and offer comfort. No emotion will be forbidden, shameful, or unsayable. Everything will be acceptable. It would also be appropriate to point out that you're not contagious and that they're in no danger, even though their fears are perfectly legitimate. Four, seven, and ten—that's young to accept ambivalence. Never mind, we're going to win. Because nothing, not even this ignominious thing, will diminish our strength as a family. We're prepared to adapt massively in order to keep your lives as close as possible to normality. Everything is different, but nothing has changed. So I establish a list of invariables for the little ones: school, friends, family, the neighborhood, and sporting and creative activities. As for the hospital, I make an asset of its nearness. It's no longer an intruder but an annex. We as a household are squaring up to the invader on its own territory and appropriating its codes. We're enlisting something that wants to take one of ours. Now we can all be together with you at the Institute whenever we like. We'll drop in on the way home from school, between the bakery and homework. We'll go there to play table soccer, to bicycle, read comic books, play piano, and sing on Wednesday afternoons or on the weekends. We'll eat in the dining room, have an after-school snack in the cafeteria, and get some fresh air in the garden. Our home is the bigger for it.

Your brother and sister like this idea. They smile and can't wait to go see you. Right now. Their energy galvanizes me. My hand makes a sudden spontaneous gesture to symbolize our resistance. First it spreads wide, and as I raise each finger I name a member of the family: thumb—Daddy; index finger—Mommy; middle finger—Solal; ring finger—Anna; little finger—Nils. Then my hand closes into a tight fist that carves powerfully, horizontally, into the air in front of me. "And a punch in the face to lymphoma!" Anna squeals jubilantly, followed by Nils, and they take turns going through the routine for themselves. They will trot it out hundreds of times and will even integrate it into a ritual dance, a secret household haka, a sign of our identity and strength. And follow it with a bellowed song that they learned goodness knows where, chanting—with remarkable intuition—Maori words that they don't even understand: *Ka mate! Ka mate! Ka ora! Ka ora!* ("'Tis death! 'Tis death! 'Tis life! 'Tis life!"). Bring it on, lymphoma. This family's invincible.

––––––––

The morning goes without a hitch: the younger two coming to the ward, the ecstatic reunion, their laughter in the corridors and the playroom. Seeing their three children together like this, Lise and Olivier could almost forget that their eldest is ill. Because the lymphoma has made itself temporarily invisible. The excrescence on his neck has disappeared, probably curbed by the first cortisone injections. Perhaps it's also to this treatment that Solal owes his particularly fresh complexion, without yet giving his face the puffiness seen in the other hospitalized children. Again unlike them, he still has his hair and can move about freely without a drip. To look at him, no one would think he was a member of the cancer community. His siblings have reclaimed him, and it feels as if they might be able to spare him his fate. He, Anna, and Nils are like three children who've come to visit someone with their parents. And when Olivier leaves to take the younger two to the recreation center, Lise practically expects him to take Solal along with them. She so wishes he would.

Less than an hour later, she is following the hospital bed on which her son lies, covered in just a white sheet, with a hygiene cap on his head. They walk through the department, pass the playroom, and take a large elevator down to the basement. Solal is very pale now. And it's not just the bluish reflection from the cap. He's frightened. Even before he gets to the treatment, he's scared of having the drip line inserted. His body has registered painful memories from Necker.

The basement is cold and impersonal. Surprisingly empty too. They go through a pair of thick double doors and then stop in a windowless room, lit by a dubious neon light. A screen stands between them and another bed. An elderly lady moans constantly. Lise tries to reassure the child. The waiting starts, never-ending. Mathilde joins them. Lise doesn't remember when. The sisters don't say much but Lise is grateful for this discreet presence by her side. A silent propinquity begins to form. A feeling of trust settles. As is often the case, Mathilde anchors her affection in her profession; it's when she uses medical terminology that she succeeds in communicating her empathy. She mentions the use of hypnosis to manage her patients' pain, and teaches her sister the rudiments of the techniques. Something is handed down, from the elder sister to the younger. For a moment Lise savors this connection, a closeness she so longed for in other circumstances and in other times. Then she puts the information into practice as she in turn hands it down to her child. It is effective and eases the dreaded insertion. Each of them now enjoys something close to serenity, until a hospital porter comes to take Solal, alone, to the operating theater. When the bed is steered into the area reserved for surgery, Solal turns to his mother and, looking her right in the eye, chirps, "Goodbye, Mommy, I'll tell you if God exists." These words are so painful to Lise that she doesn't even realize it. In fact, she doesn't know what to make of them. Humor already constitutes a form of resistance for her son. So she's not sure whether he's joking or serious. Either way, she's well aware that a quip like this can't possibly be neutral. There's too much panache in its derision. What internal crisis is the child presenting with these words? Is he even aware how brutal they are? Once Lise had reminded him this procedure was harmless, it seems the last thing she said to him, with a forced smile, was, "What nonsense. You talk complete nonsense." She thinks she remembers that, the moment the bed was wheeled out of sight, she caught her sister's eye and looked for her shoulder so she could rest her head, sobbing. She also thinks she remembers that Mathilde—for the first time—put her arms around her, with tears in her eyes.

At 2 p.m. Lise and Olivier are alone at home. It's a good three hours since their son went into theater. He's having a triple procedure: the insertion of the port-a-cath, followed by a lumbar puncture to take cerebrospinal fluid and inject the first dose of chemotherapy. The parents wait anxiously to be called. They can't really think how to kill the time. The phone rings at last: everything went well and Solal is in the recovery room. This is more than just relief, it's happiness itself. They set off immediately to be by his side, hurrying and full of smiles. They could almost run, allowing themselves to be carried by an elementary syllogism: the treatment has started, and this treatment is meant to cure Solal, therefore Solal is on

the way to being cured. As if having successfully overcome a
first obstacle has taken them straight to victory, ignoring the
intervening stages. So, blithe and lighthearted, they walk up
rue Claude-Bernard hand in hand. Blithe and lighthearted,
they enter the Institute and go down to the basement. Still
blithe and lighthearted, they lose their way in the corridors
and, without realizing it, end up at the entrance to the operating area. Lastly, blithe and lighthearted, they come across a
doctor. A tall, rangy man. All they can see of him are his eyes;
everything else is swallowed up by his scrubs: hood, mask,
tunic, pants, and steel blue overshoes. The man starts by rep-
rimanding them; they're not allowed in this area without permission. Still not shaking off their buoyant mood, the parents
explain that they're looking for the recovery room where their
son is. They're in the right place: the man's an anesthetist and
has in fact just been on hand for Solal's operation. "So he's
fine, then," the parents say enthusiastically. They can't wait to
celebrate the good news with one of the contributors to this success. It's their own private national holiday, their miniature
liberation. Bring out the flags, climb the barricades, clam-
ber over tanks, sing and dance. Of course, some small part
of them knows—all too clearly—that the war is not yet won.
That this wasn't even a true battle. More a case of lining up
the troops. But hope needs to withdraw to this moment, as if it
were everything. To concentrate its forces on it. To make of it a
solid kernel that can radiate all the energy needed to confront
what is to come. In fact, they're quite determined never to miss

an opportunity for celebration. The anesthetist, meanwhile, does not see it like this. Is he amazed by their detachment, outraged by their high spirits, tired from his day's work, or slightly obtuse? In any event, he chooses not to spare them. He lifts his arms to chest height, holds his hands about eight inches apart, and keeps them firmly in position around some unidentified object while he snaps back, "Don't be too quick to celebrate. I've just come from his op and I saw the tumor. Your son is far from cured. There's a risk it won't work. It's not looking good. It's a huge mass, you know, this big." Not as huge, though, Lise thinks straightaway, as the blow you've just dealt us. Because they'll have to cope with this now. With these words and, more important, that gesture. An indecent gesture that gave the thing a size, a shape, a tangibility. An obscene gesture that implied the outline of the invisible. They've met the man who's seen, the man who's plumbed the intimate depths of the disease. And this man's hands are illustrating how serious it is while his words condemn their hope. The parents must have an extra serving of illusion and obstinacy, and perhaps a hint of arrogance, because they simply reply, "We'll see. For now we're glad the procedure's done and we just want to see him."

It's the afternoon and you're back in your room. I don't remember what you were like that day. Not at all. Are you still half-asleep? Do your scars hurt? Are you relieved you didn't get to see whether God exists? I'd love to say we laughed about that with hindsight. But I've forgotten. On the other hand, I do remember someone coming to find us, your father and me, for another meeting with the oncologist. This time the meeting is held in the "parents' room." A small, quiet space set apart within the outpatient department, where people can take refuge should the need arise to read, think, or weep. Efforts have been made to make the room relaxing, with small sofas, a coffee table, and magazines. The décor, with its halfhearted nautical theme, apparently wants to encourage daydreaming. In actual fact, I find the porthole window in the door, the blue and yellow leatherette furniture, and the pictures of dolphins no more conducive to dreaming than the linoleum floor, the hygiene advice all over the walls, and the persistent smell of antiseptics. The space is at least more intimate than a consulting room. This second meeting certainly marks further familiarity with the medical team. We come in to find Dr. O, and sit ourselves around the coffee table with him. We're given a glass of water. The place is nice but also slightly laughable. First, because the furniture is far too small for the doctor and your father, who have to fold their limbs awkwardly to sit down. Alice in the white rabbit's house, Gulliver in Lilliput. There's something deliciously childish about it that subtly amuses me. But my private humor is also, if not black, at least defensive. I do realize that this comfortable atmosphere is fallacious. Painful memories

IF

of the first meeting are still drilled into my body, and, although I don't understand the need for this rerun, I'm afraid
of it. The deliberate warmth chills me, particularly as—just
like the day before—we're flanked by nurses. Petite women
who certainly belong more in this space than the doctor.
But I find their silence disturbing. I now know they're definitely here to catch us should we collapse. And, strangely,
knowing this safety net is there is oppressive rather than reassuring. As if being protected generates danger. So, in the
hope of self-preservation, I'm amused by this discrepancy,
smile ironically at the awkwardness of the situation, stray-
ing ever further from my true feelings. Reality soon catches
up with me. This meeting is indeed an agonizing rerun. It
is intended precisely to reiterate everything we were told
the day before, facts that they assume—quite rightly—we
weren't able to assimilate. Reiterating them but in more
detail. A painstaking breakdown of the protocol, stage by
stage, including the problems, risks, and side effects. The
configuration of the room facilitates the educational aspect
of the conversation. Dr. O has put a sheet of paper and a
pen on the coffee table. He marks out the chronology of the
months ahead. Our lives boil down to this arrow pointing
toward an uncertain future. Somewhere to the right, beyond the page, the target is reached. Or missed. The outcome remains unresolved. Meanwhile, the stages along the
way are clearly defined. They are represented by vertical
lines that punctuate the graduated scale. Your stations of

the cross. This graphic representation isn't eloquent enough and needs to be reinforced with commentary. This time I understand everything. In other words, they were right to start over. I ask questions, register information, file facts. My vocabulary grows: aplasia, alopecia, protocol, parenteral, polynuclear, neutrophils, neutropenia, lymphocyte, mucositis, myelogram, lumbar puncture, septicemia, stomatitis, thrombocytopenia. Acronyms pop up all over the place: PAC, PET, PHP, GMC, ANC, WBC, CBC, FBE, IV. And the letters are soon joined by numbers. They accumulate on the sheet of paper, under the time arrow. Your illness is also a math study, part counts, part statistics. The potential figures for your white blood cells are spelled out before my eyes in black and white, and in reverse order: the normal levels you will no longer achieve, the minimal threshold needed for you to cope with chemo sessions, the zero point that you will head toward again and again. Because the linearity of this diagram is deceptive. Your actual trajectory will be disjointed. It will unfold vertically, a sawtooth line, from top to bottom and bottom to top, with each aplasia. Every course of chemo will reduce your defenses to nothing and we will have to wait for the levels to rally before starting the next. And medicine can do nothing to combat this. Only your body, your personal stamina, will determine how long it takes. We grasp, between the lines, that it is here, in the places where the growth curve of your neutrophils is inverted, that your survival will play out.

And you will have only a short window every time. Skulking in the shadows, the lymphoma will need only a brief respite to gather its strength again. So we are still goaded by the urgency of the first two days. Even then, obviously the protocol needs to work. Sometimes, we're told, the cancerous cells withstand it. Then different molecules must be tried, until the right ones are identified. What if? What if they're not identified? I don't ask. I know the answer.

Even though the teaching methods are better today, the effect produced is no different from yesterday. The rigorous methodical approach proves equally devastating. I now understand it so completely that it soon becomes unbearable. All the same, I cling on for a moment, trying to elicit more encouraging answers. To achieve this, I go back to the more reassuring linear diagram and infiltrate the gaps. I insert the omissions and put meaning into the line's sloping edges, before and after each gradation, in the places where there should apparently be no difficulties. I ask a succession of questions that aspire to be statements:

"So my son will be hospitalized for a whole week every three weeks, but that means he'll be home for the other two weeks?" "Actually, no. Because after a couple of days"—the pen draws another vertical line—"when he's in total aplasia, he's bound to catch an infection. So we'll need to monitor his temperature and will have to bring it down within the hour as soon as it goes above one hundred degrees to avoid septicemia. Don't worry, we know how to manage it."

"But once the infection is over, he can come home?" "Actually, no. Because this will usually coincide with when he's recovering from aplasia and the start of the next round of chemotherapy"—the pen goes over old lines, making them thicker.

"Solal will hardly eat anything while the treatment is going on because of the vomiting, so, as I understand it, he'll be fed intravenously, but he'll catch up between sessions? He'll get his appetite back?" "Actually, no. Because the aplasia will go hand in hand with ulcers all over his mouth, so he won't tolerate contact with food at all. So we're likely to resort to artificial feeding a lot of the time. Don't worry, we know how to manage that."

"Solal will at least be able to have a good time in the playroom and follow regular lessons in the inpatient classroom?" "Actually, no. The type of chemo he's having is particularly aggressive because his cancer spreads very quickly, so he won't have much strength, especially in the first two months. You really mustn't hope he'll be able to concentrate on anything else."

Silly me with my illusions. The disjointed line has caught up with me and even I am starting to flag in its successive ups and downs. My stomach hurts and I feel hotter and hotter. The size of the room doesn't help. Any more than your father's and the doctor's physical discomfort, or being flanked by the two nurses. The walls draw closer, the space shrinks, oxygen becomes scarce. Anxiety squeezes in on me, clutches at my throat. I snap, somewhere between mucositis and lumbar punctures. As I did the day before, I urgently need to remove myself from what Dr. O is saying. Yesterday my skin was being attacked; today it's my flesh. I ask to leave the room. I beg them to excuse me, saying I need to get some air.

As I come back into the room I catch the end of a sentence: "...but we won't know that till he reaches puberty." No point elaborating on what they're discussing. I understand and I have no interest in it. Confronted with the accumulation of immediate dangers, potential sterility in the future feels like a very secondary problem. So I bounce back smugly on that last word. "Puberty...well, at least that means he'll be alive." The rest really doesn't matter. "So," Dr. O says, picking up the piece of paper again, "this is the short protocol if everything goes to plan. Except we don't yet have confirmation of the exact stage of the cancer. We won't know that till Friday, when we have the results of the in-depth tests. The lymphoma could still become leukemia, because if the cancer has gotten into his cerebrospinal fluid—remember we took a sample of that during this morning's procedure—we'll have to implement a protocol that's twice as long and more complex." With a prognosis, I can't help thinking, that's twice as grim. "Let me explain." "No thank you, Dr. O." The words just slipped out. I smile and temper this abrupt refusal with a few polite but no less ironic sentences: "Allow me to decline that offer. We already have enough information. If you don't mind, we'll leave it there to start with and we'll hear the longer version if and when we need to. That's enough for today." The doctor nods. I think he's tired of this conversation too. I do have one last question for him, though. It relates to the size of the thing. I describe our meeting with the anesthetist and the fears it sparked. The doctor reminds us that with lymphoma it's not appropriate to focus on one particular tumor. It's more to do with how far it's spread through the whole lymphatic system and particularly in the fluid around the brain and spinal cord. In fact, that's why the treatment is administered into the blood rather than with surgery. Surprising though it may seem, I find this answer reassuring. That mass can swell all it likes. I'm happier with growth than spreading. I'd be only too glad to hear that his lymphoma has parked itself in his tonsil, however monstrous it is. The important thing now is dispersal. Before letting us go the doctor adds, "In future, if you want to know how a patient is numbed, ask an anesthetist. But if your question is about cancer, it's better to ask an oncologist." This time Dr. O can leave satisfied: he managed to tell us the worst, he gave us fresh hope, and, in the end, he made me laugh.

The parents barely have time to dwell on what the doctor has told them, because they need to leave right away. On this the last Wednesday before the Christmas holidays they're meant to be watching their daughter Anna's dance show. They didn't want to cancel it. So many things are about to change for their family that, right from the start, they want to leave in place anything that can be left. Still, it feels strange finding themselves in this gym surrounded by carefree parents and ebullient children less than an hour after their meeting with the oncologist. They're torn in two. One part of them has stayed at the Institute, the other is trying to keep going in the outside world. Saying hello to some people, smiling from a distance to others, keeping quiet, most of all keeping quiet. On the stage vigorous childish bodies move about freely. Latin music, red flounces, tango steps. The emotion is intense, well nigh unbearable. Olivier is filming. Lise sits hugging Nils close and desperately holding eye contact with Anna. Her daughter is now the only thing she sees, and she tries, in vain, to succumb to the delights of her dancing.

5

Two large metal pincers grab a six-inch oblong glass tube filled with transparent liquid. A technician wearing a thick green apron carries it at arm's length over to a small cubicle surrounded by curtains. He sets the tube into a receptacle hanging from an IV pole with several pipes connected to a child lying on a bed. The place is dark, bathed in a strange bluish light. Lise can barely make out her own son in the shadows, but he's definitely there, ready to have the injection of radioactive fluid in preparation for his PET scan. This examination is part of the research protocol in which she and Olivier agreed to participate the day before. During their meeting in the "parents' room" the oncologist suggested adding this new type of investigation to the usual scans. He gave a rundown of the advantages, chiefly its greater accuracy in identifying cancerous cells. He also put forward another, irresistible argument: without clinical trials like this, without the consent of other parents in other research programs, the treatment that their son is about to undergo would take twice as long with twice as many side effects to achieve a similar result. He then handed them a booklet describing the aims of the research, how it was being carried out, the treatment and monitoring of patients participating in the trials, but also risk management and undesirable or unexpected effects associated with the trial. He asked them to read it and sign it promptly if they agreed to the procedure. Overwhelmed by the accumulation of oral information, the parents didn't have it in them to read the booklet. Lise simply asked the oncologist to summarize why, given the apparently irrefutable aid to recovery offered by this test, anyone would be tempted to refuse it. That was when Dr. O mentioned the use of radioactive substances that, even though used in doses that were no threat to health, might put some people off. The parents concluded this was no time for dithering and signed the document on the spot. Now that it is a reality, though, Lise is wondering just how innocuous the test is. Is this due to the precautions taken by the technician to protect himself? Or the meticulous protocol set up to keep her safe herself? She has been seated more than three feet from her son, so that she's unable to hold his hand—quite an achievement, given the size of the cubicle. Then a mobile lead screen topped with a glass window has been installed in front of her, and she's been told to stay behind it and not to move. Lastly a dosimeter, a sort of miniature Geiger counter, has been attached to the back of her jacket, and it emits its crackling sound if she leans one way or the other behind her shield. Definitely no danger, then. For her at least. The atmosphere needs relaxing.

Solal must stay still for a couple of hours while the reactive material diffuses through his body. But he is allowed to talk. After giving him a few explanations about the test, Lise points to the glass tube: "It is quite big for a suppository, but don't worry, it won't hurt!" Mother and son laugh out loud. Then they both drift into a half sleep, lulled by the blink of neon lights and the regular rasp of the drip pump. Two hours later Solal has his PET scan. The scanner should provide a more accurate representation of the spread of the disease. They will be given the results the following day.

The day drags on in your hospital room. Your father left early this morning, before the PET scan, to give Anna and Nils a kiss before catching a few hours' rest at home. He had a disrupted night with you: you slept badly and woke many times complaining of sharp pains in your back and head, probably a consequence of the previous day's procedure, your first lumbar puncture and the injection of chemotherapeutic agents into your cerebrospinal fluid. I wasn't there at the time to soothe you, cradle you, and reassure you. I wasn't there by your side if you needed me. It's unbearable. Still, I do now have to accept that I can't be with you when I'm looking after your brother and sister, and I can't be with them when I'm looking after you. Your hospitalization has sliced up my strength and torn to pieces

my ties. On this front, as a couple, the fact that there are
two of us at least gives powerless parents a sense of ubiq-
uity. Right from the start your father automatically took on
the nights at the Institute and I the days. We didn't discuss it, we didn't make a decision about it, that's just what
happened. Only much later will I understand it is the one
possible solution. I'm probably already intuitively aware
why. I genuinely wouldn't cope with what Olivier is going
through: sleeping badly, for a start, on an uncomfortable
cot at your feet in a room shared with another sick child and
another parent on another cot. Constantly woken by alarms
on pumps, by the comings and goings of nurses changing
over chemo pouches, by snoring, cries of pain, and calls for
help. Like a sailor's sleep, light and fragmented, but your
father then needs to emerge bright-eyed and bushy-tailed to
take on the day. With no shower, no wash, no privacy. And
not for just one night, or two, but for dozens and dozens of
consecutive nights. You father has his own inner peace; he
knows how to shut things out and ignore the bustle of the
outside world to get to sleep and recharge his batteries. He's
a marathon runner, he has a strong constitution and the
endurance to face any ordeal. But to be honest, more than
these numerous problems, what I couldn't bear is missing
out on things as Olivier does: not taking the other two to
school, not kissing them goodnight in bed, not being there
when they're frightened in the night or struggling to get
up in the morning. And then not helping you through all

your tests, not meeting the people you talk to, not sharing in your languid days, not living in your world. I want to experience the horrors inflicted on you firsthand, to look them in the eye and stand up to them in the fight. I want to ease your every pain, take on the weight of your suffering, make a shield of my body and a rampart of my mind. Given that I can't take your place, I will be a decoy, inviting the enemy to change its target. I don't sleep next to you, but I shall keep constant watch over you with my eyes wide open. Conversely, your father feels no frustration at not being here during the day, because it's the difficulties of the daytime activities that he wouldn't be able to tolerate. He doesn't have my medical heritage; he doesn't benefit from this specific acclimatization to the hospital's codes that constitutes a sort of desensitization. He is in fact extremely vulnerable. He pales at the least mention of physical pain, feels nauseous from the smell of antiseptics, and swoons at the sight of a syringe. When he has a blood test he gets so tense that his veins contract and the blood won't flow. He is well aware how detrimental this weakness of his could be to you. The nighttime darkness, combined with the relative slowing in medical activity while you sleep, suits him better. He'll protect you with his eyes closed, in silence and in the dark. And so for months on end, and perhaps more, I will be wherever your father is not, and he will be wherever I'm not. Our personality differences will serve us well. Between us we will hold on tight to the ends of the rope so that, although apart, we can keep the family circle together. Mind you, what will be left of us as a couple afterward? I don't think about this for now. It's not the time. The most important thing is that you never feel alone.

The division of tasks between your father and me may have happened spontaneously from the outset, but an objective factor soon validates it: as a civil servant, I can stop work for some time without the risk of losing my job, whereas your father, who works in the private sector, can't. Yes, the outside world does keep on turning. While we're fighting for your life we do still, rather more prosaically, need to keep the family alive. You see, illness isn't satisfied with devastating bodies and hearts; it also entails an endless retinue of material problems. We haven't yet thought about that; it seems such a minor concern. But we understand the scope of it on this fourth day when we meet the social worker.

Sarah Liguri is a young, very straightforward-looking woman. She sees us in her office in the outpatient department. Jeans, baggy sweater, hair loosely held in a messy bun, she is kind and direct. Her relaxed appearance, fresh face, and kindness are a stark contrast with the harsh administrative realities for which she is responsible. She is in fact in a very tricky position. She meets people cloaked in brand-new agony, people who have no interest in the demands of the real world, and has to hand them additional concerns. She is the conduit for this double hit. Granted, she presents herself as attorney for labor law, guiding us through countless processes that will help protect our financial circumstances: arranging for 100 percent of your medical costs to be paid plus the daily hospital fees, reimbursing our transport costs, an 80 percent invalidity card, and a variety of work leaves and allocations offered to parents so that they can be with their sick child. The wonders of the French social system. But at the same time Sarah has to point out to us the system's limitations. Admirable it may indeed be, but it's not enough. How could it be? As the oncologist warned us when we very first arrived, the brutality of your treatment means both parents will be needed all the time. So we'll both have to stop working, but we'd still want to be—quite legitimately—paid at the same rate and be allowed to reclaim our respective jobs afterward. We the spoiled children of this republic discover to our amazement that our loss of employment won't be compensated for with sums that match our salaries. Not even close. Thanks to the AJPP, the French daily allocation for parental attendance, Sarah explains gently, we're each entitled to a flat-rate allowance of 41.17 euros a day for 22 days every month, for a maximum of 310 days. That doesn't even cover the cost of our rent. It's not enough to live properly. What if? What if you're sick for more than 310 days? Then we'd have nothing. It's a harsh blow. There is, however, one possibility for complementary help. The social worker suddenly looks embarrassed when she refers to it. She only mentions it, she says, in the absence of any other solution and when a long and complicated application needs to be put together and implemented as quickly as possible. But she's afraid she'll distress us and, before naming the option, reminds us that because you have cancer you're entitled to be recognized as incapacitated. For a moment I wonder what this taboo word, this unutterable aspect of your illness, can be. I can think of only one and it's definitely not that, so I encourage her to speak freely. She then tells us about the allocation of funds for the education of disabled children, a monthly sum of 124.54 euros guaranteed by the French "disability law" of February 11, 2005. "Disabled," is that the no-no in our vocabulary? I don't understand and put the question to Sarah. The thing is, she says, some parents refuse this allowance simply because of the word, they're ashamed of it. I can't see the logic myself. After all, what does it matter if it's disability, invalidity, incapacity, or cancer? All that any of them means is bad luck. The debasement is due to the facts, not the word. To tell the truth, faced with this financial stalemate, I'm hardly at my leisure to linger over these semantic distinctions. They can call their file whatever they like, so long as they give me enough for my family to live on. My ethics relax at the same time as my semantic rigor. Most likely this too is partly a secret rebellion. Confronted with the scandalous injustice of your illness, I'm looking for some form of compensation. And as such I'm not above a minor abuse of language. So "Disabled" you shall be. Is it my sudden flexibility that encourages Sarah to confide in us with one last option, on the very limits of legitimacy, or does she suggest it systematically to all parents? It is, quite simply, for us to ask our own doctors for sickness leave. The grounds cited in these cases, Sarah informs us, are post-traumatic depression. "But I'm not sick. How can I be entitled to that? I won't take it." My superego is balking at this. Anyway, my moral reasoning adds almost desperately, what with no vacations, no trips, no outings, and no activities, we'll hardly need any money. It will take a few weeks for me to change my mind. Long enough for me to understand that, without my salary, Anna's and Nils's lives are shockingly diminished. Long enough also for me to acknowledge that even though in the heat of the moment I may be impregnable, somewhere deep down this trauma is silently gnawing at my fragile foundations.

The meeting with the social worker lasts more than an hour and introduces the parents to a tortuously convoluted world. They have a glimpse of the difficult steps taken by thousands of other parents of sick or disabled children. They expand their collection of glossy brochures and soon rack up a new list of acronyms: HAD, PAI, ALD, AEEH, VSL, AJPP,

APAESIC, MDPH, CDAPH, SAPAD, SFCE, UNAPE-CLE. They fill in dozens of pages of forms, estimating the cost of Solal's illness in euros. Loss of employment, need for family support, private transport—their fight is translated into expenses and loss of earnings. Where do they find the motivation to do all this, barely four days after the first shock and before the enemy has even been wholly identified? They should be gripped, paralyzed, by a phobia of administration. The whole thing should turn their stomachs: the forms with their boxes to fill in, the leaflets with their sclerotic pronouncements, the precisely dated laws and decrees, the allowances defined down to the last cent, the percentages and the calculations. One hundred percent of medical costs paid, invalidity at 80 percent, 30 percent reduction, 20 percent markup, 10 percent mitigation, three days' leave, five days', three months', 41.17-euro allowance per day, 22 days a month, 310 days per illness, 49 euros a day for three weeks, 124.54 euros per month per disability, 93.41 euros supplemented for category 1, 252.98 for category 2, 358.06 for category 3, 554.88 for category 4, 709.16 for category 5, and 1,029.10 for category 6, in keeping with the laws of July 25, 1994, August 21, 2003, February 11, 2005, December 19, 2005, and December 21, 2006. They are forced to quantify things that, by definition, are beyond all calculation. An unendurable inventory of despair. The figures proliferate before their eyes at the same rate as their son's deranged cells. They become familiar with the stereotyped formulae of legislative jargon that deftly articulate descriptions, injunctions, and conditions. It is allocated, it is paid, it is guaranteed, it is renewed, you will receive. You will need to prove, you will inform, the doctor must certify, the employer must accept. Under certain conditions, if the child is younger than twelve months, if he/she is younger than twenty, if he/ she is in a specialized establishment, if he/she is more than 80 percent disabled, if there are at least three dependents, if you have been in your present employment for one year, thirty-six months, six years, if you are an undocumented immigrant, if you live alone, if you have no social cover, if you have no resources. If. So many restrictions on something so random.

After a while the mother seems to switch off. She plays a mental game, combining words and figures to create outlandish combinations: "According to the law of April 137, '05, you will be allocated 22.1 categories of the discounted third disability for a period of 94.41 workdays, for a maximum of 4.2 cancers of the same type, if you do not exceed 9 percent of the funding ceiling established on blabla 36, 1912, or if you live alone with more than 3.01 dependent children aged less than one, on condition that you can prove that you have had a day job and a night job as an undocumented immigrant for a minimum of twelve years. Or if you don't understand any of it." This parody affords the mother some relief for a time. She can't be bothered with these forms, the terms are too definite, the numbers too finite, and the boxes too small for her to house her pain. And yet she knows she needs to play along. She understands how import-ant this is, even though she may not feel it.

Despite the incongruity of the process, Lise and Olivier succeed, without unnecessary stress or hesitation, in establishing a definitive hierarchy of their needs and in making the correct choices. Looking back, they will be amazed they managed it. Only then will they understand the vital role played by the young woman who walked them through this task: she accepted their distress; she introduced empathy into the very arid terrain of administrative discourse; she imbued the numbers with their qualitative meaning. Her apparent simplicity harbored tremendous delicacy. Something more than professionalism. Humanity. Perhaps for the first time, as they emerged from this meeting, the parents seemed calm.

Lise is sitting on the bench in the corridor, facing the piano. Her son is asleep in the nearby room. What can she be thinking about right now? Her horizons have shrunk. She can neither think about the events of the last few days (too traumatic) nor envisage the months to come (too frightening) nor dream about what might have been (too painful). So, quite naturally, she sticks to the present. First, she watches passersby, then, when they have stopped passing by, she focuses her attention on things. She is particularly interested in a mark on the linoleum. It has an animal-like shape, somewhere between a horse and a llama. Lise studies it for a long time, then scrutinizes the rest of the floor in search of other chimeras. Her reverie is interrupted when a woman comes to sit next to her. It's the mother of the little girl who shares Solal's room, and her name is Lyudmyla. She's Ukrainian. At first she looks Lise directly in the eye, as if transmitting a silent message. Then she talks to her, in English, about her daughter. Luba is five. She has a bone sarcoma and has been having treatment at the Institute for three months. She's bald, very thin and pale. Lyudmyla segues seamlessly into asking Lise a series of questions in a disconcertingly procedural tone of voice: "Are you French?" "Yes." "Do you work here in France?" "Yes, I'm a lecturer." "How long have you been working in this country?" "About fifteen years." "So you've paid taxes all that time, haven't you?" "Ye...es." A Ukrainian tax inspector in the middle of the Curie, that's as entertaining as a horse-llama. Even so, Lise is starting to wonder what this interrogation is about when Lyudmyla suddenly grabs her hand and, shaking her arm, mutters quietly, "Thank you. Thank you for saving my daughter." Her voice cracks with emotion. She has tears in her eyes. Lise doesn't immediately understand. However kindly disposed she may be toward Luba, her main impression was that the little girl's video game made far too much noise. She doesn't really see how this could save the child. Besides, she doesn't grasp the coherence of this conversation that has unexpectedly changed flavor, switching abruptly from taxes to survival. She asks for an explanation. The thing is, the young woman explains in English, every foreign child whose cancer can't be treated in his or her country of origin is offered chemotherapy in France. A dual inheritance from France's so-cial system and its tradition as a place of refuge, made possi-ble by the fact that it maintains its public services. Hospital, in the etymological sense of the word. Lise should love this. Every aspect of it corresponds not only with her convictions but, more privately still, with the very role she has always felt she was meant to play. A late-born accident in a chaotic family environment, she is the swan song for imperiled desire. Origins like that bind you firmly to an indissoluble mission. For as long as she can remember, and wherever she has been, Lise has, by some disturbing automatic process, found herself in a tutelary role. Concern, listening, and support form the basis for all her energy. She takes the word "sympathy" lit-erally and, creating an indigestible concoction, combines the self-abnegation of a scapegoat, the hypersensitivity of a pre-cocious child, a moral obsession with fulfilling duties, and the enthusiastic ambition of a redeemer. And the whole package is haunted by the specter of failure. Aware of her own flaws, Lise is therefore amazed to find she isn't awash with emotion. It's such a beautiful moment: a mother's tears and gratitude, the communion of two suffering souls at the bedsides of their ailing children, a frail creature saved by an effective collective system, a foreigner taken in, tended, perhaps cured, illness transcended and overcome in an act of reciprocation. Anyone would think it was a movie. Zoom in on these two careworn faces, these misty eyes, these interwoven fingers; musical crescendo accompanying an epiphanic smile, the fervor of a maternal eucharist and the sublimation of evil. All the factors have come together for extraordinary transports of emotion. But nothing. As if detached from herself, Lise watches the scene without experiencing the expected resonance from it. Yes, she squeezes Lyudmyla's hands in return and looks her kindly in the eye. Her eyes even fill with tears. But she feels deep down she is lying. She tries to gauge her imposture and, not without shame, notes the orderly sequence of her first prosaic, selfish, mean-spirited thoughts. "Saving foreign children at public expense is obviously a good thing. But it might have been a good idea, first, to consider letting us be at our son's bedside without ruining us and breaking up our family. We don't even get a single room, for a start..." A thought that is despised, regretted, and atoned for almost before it is acknowledged. Incredible, Lise thinks, how hardship can produce a knee-jerk nationalism. She'll have to watch out for that. This nightmare will soon make a protectionist of her. As she plumbs the depths of self-loathing, she does have to confess that, right now, Luba's life doesn't matter that much to her. She can think only of her own loved ones. Solal, Anna, and Nils are her exclusive priorities. It's about saving energy. She knows she's inclined to take on other people's problems and is afraid of being contaminated by their pain. Convinced that, this time, she doesn't have the strength for everything, she decides to get her priorities straight and ignore anything, whatever it may be, inessential to her family. And so for many long weeks, as she focuses on her battle, this mother who is usually so sociable will make a point of avoiding any kind of personal conversation and will deliberately confine herself to superficial exchanges with the other parents and their sick children.

This day that started so anxiously eventually brings me to my most private hopes. At least that's what I believe in the tiny leeway of freedom left to me by this lymphoma. As I did at home in the bath a couple of evenings ago, but this time on a bench seat in the corridor of the Institute that has become peculiarly familiar, I feel centered. Resolute in my choices, determined in my actions. Until this afternoon, I thought I could continue working. I teach at the university in Grenoble and had pictured myself juggling between seminars, high-speed trains, chemo sessions, and lumbar punctures. I went to great lengths to find illusory practical solutions, shrugging off the 370 miles between here and my place of work. I conjured up working models, constructed strategies. It has to be said I'm a seasoned expert: having had this job for eight years, I've had to reexamine my schedule and my motives with each of my younger two children's births. As my hopes for a transfer shrank with the decline in university humanities departments, I've had to make the best of this split life. The geographical distance, the nights in hotels, the uncertainties, and the delayed trains. It's been grueling, to say the least, but it still held, at the cost of many sacrifices, until you became sick. And here I am this evening grasping the fact that I no longer have the option of going back to work. Your cancer makes it impossible. It may seem restrictive but I'm relieved that my own wishes have had to bow to the pressing needs of the real world. I can almost convince myself I'm glad I have to stop work. Any more and I'll be indebted to this lymphoma. I'm bested by my own best arguments. They contrive a perverse logic, causing me to pretend I'm choosing what has been thrust upon me. Now I can see only the inconveniences of my former circumstances. I forget the structuring qualities, ignore the social virtues, and underestimate the intellectual benefits. I don't need that anymore. I've found another job.

So I won't be going back to the university. I'll be by your side every day, all day long. You'll never be abandoned to your pain, needs, or anxiety. You can offload your aches and fears, your rages and tears onto me. And on the tiniest parcel of hope, I'll build you a whole world of laughter and things you want. I'll counter the machines that are going to exhaust your bodily functions and drain your vitality. I'll give you a transfusion of all my strength and the will to fight. I'll give you a lust for life. But if you collapse, if there's not the smallest spark left, well, then I'll open my arms to accept your despair. Because more than anything else I want you to stay completely true to yourself. I will be merely a support. You will be sick and in pain but you alone will be at the controls of your fate. To achieve this I'll have

to invent a respectful presence by your side, one that is both
solid and permeable, loyal and transparent.

Bolstered by these resolutions, I go to see the child psychiatrist who has given me my first appointment at the end
of the afternoon. Dr. Seigneur (Dr. Lord!) has such a pre-
destined name that it could be a witticism. Is this about
ensuring that these children whose lives are threatened
have some first contact with the impenetrable ways of the
divine? In the vast mediatized confessional of our atheist
society, haven't psychiatrists taken on the priest's former
role, listening, guiding, absolving, and sometimes appor-
tioning blame? When I'm told his name all I hear initially
are biblical echoes. And yes, he may not be the messiah,
but he's at least one of the forms of support on which I'm
depending to help you come through this ordeal. He will
listen, in privacy, to your suffering, allow you to confess
the unspeakable, deliver you of your silences. He will have
access to the things I don't notice, to all the things a mother
doesn't see and hear, to everything she cannot and must
not know. He will be able to mitigate my shortcomings and
remedy my mistakes.

We talk about you, about these early days, the first
pain, the diagnosis, and how we were informed. We mention the future. Then he asks me how I am. I'm surprised,

bordering on offended. I feel as if I'm impinging on your territory. "I'm very well, thank you. But I thought you were a child psychiatrist, so that's not really the question." "True, I'm a child psychiatrist," he replies calmly, "but surely looking after children also means listening to their parents?" Dr. Seigneur has a very distinctive way of speaking—slowly, clearly enunciated but also vigorous. There is a sense of constrained gravity, as if the apparent simplicity of his questions disguises unfathomable depths. As if he were condensing infinite digressions and reticulated revelations in a few tight-knit words and a few sibylline nods of the head. At first I'm not sure whether this is shyness or a considered professional approach. I soon tend toward the second option. And at the same time I discover other, less amusing connotations to the man's name. A lord can of course be oppressive and merciless. Maieutics can have the precision of a scalpel. It doesn't take me long to realize that I won't come out of this so well because, while I stubbornly insist that I'm absolutely fine and that I personally don't need anything, the doctor sets to work on helping me acknowledge my true feelings. Apparently going along wholeheartedly with my claims, he explores another access point. "So why don't you tell me how it all started." It's a simple request. If he wants the story, I can give it to him. I embark on it with a degree of assurance, because I'm talking about you. But then I get to the first evening of your illness, and it is at this point I realize to my astonishment that twenty-four hours of my life have vanished from my memory. The early part of your hospitalization has gone. The silence in my brain freezes me for a moment. Then I retrace my narrative a few hours and, using this as a run-up, I launch myself a second time into describing our arrival at Necker. I try again, starting from an earlier point. Same thing. I wait awhile, then strike out of the blue straight at the gaping void, thinking I might take the memory by surprise. In vain. There's definitely nothing I can do about it. In the end I'm intrigued by this adventure. I've never experienced a blackout like this before. In some ways it appeals to me; I'm fascinated by the powers of the subconscious. I smile at Dr. Seigneur. "You were right, you see. I must actually not be okay. It's just I don't know it." It will take many further sessions for me to experience my heartbreak at last. For me to cry. When I go home that evening I do at least know that somewhere inside me I'm so terribly wounded that I've had to forget it.

6

Friday, December 21. Day Five.

*When will they ever be given back their child? Two days ago,
Lise hoped with all her might that the hospital would keep him
in as long as possible. She felt ill-equipped to face the accumulation of suffering and risk produced by his chemotherapy. But
now, waking this morning, she's overwhelmed by an unbearable
feeling of loss. Her son has been taken from her, suddenly, with
no warning. It's an abduction, a kidnapping. Child snatchers!
She's amazed to be having such a primitive reaction. No one
has actually told them when this first phase will be over, but
Lise knows this is because the decision hangs on the results of
the in-depth tests. And they are to be announced this morning.
Behind her son's absence lurks fear; terrible, despotic, gnawing
fear. In the hours to come she will put on different faces, invent-
ing masks so as not to show herself. First she displays withdrawal
symptoms: aching muscles, nausea, jumpiness, and irritability.
She paces endlessly, reeling and drifting, unable to sit down for
a moment. Then she is overrun by uncontrollable thoughts that
monopolize her mind. Probably a way to fill the emptiness in*

there. Initially haphazard, they gradually come together into a dense weft and warp through which the shuttle of her distress plies secretly back and forth. One first thread takes her back three weeks to the office of the pediatrician who's been caring for her three children for several years. Solal had a sore throat and had been tired for a few days. One of his tonsils, just one, was abnormally enlarged and red, with white spots. Definite signs of tonsillitis. Lise waited to have the bacterial infection confirmed, but the swab dipped into a pipette of reactive liquid refuted it. The pediatrician concluded that it must be a virus and they must simply wait for it to heal on its own. Lise felt uncomfortable with this diagnosis. She couldn't understand how a virus could distend just one of Solal's twin tonsils so out of proportion, while leaving the other looking perfectly normal. This imbalance worried her. There was no logic to it. She admitted as much to the pediatrician, who made an ironic comment about mothers and their alarmist tendencies, then reiterated her diagnosis. So mother and son left, waiting for the promised recovery, while the villainous enemy advanced unimpeded. And now, as she waits for today's fateful results, this memory surfaces and, freighted with apprehension, swells. Soon it takes every inch of space, locking down access to her powers of reason, saturating her thoughts. Lise feels that if, during those two weeks when she abided by the pediatrician's incorrect opinion, the lymphoma progressed from stage two to stage three, making the most of the misdiagnosis to invade her son's cerebrospinal fluid and halving his chances of survival, she would never, but never forgive the woman. She feels new emotions washing over her, emotions she doesn't immediately recognize although she experiences their terrible virulence. Hate, resentment, and anger grow inside her as she weaves tirelessly back and forth through those two weeks abandoned to cancerous proliferation. It becomes so obsessive that Lise eventually substitutes herself for the subject in question, to the extent that she feels the only thing she now fears is her own violent loathing of the pediatrician. She almost gets to the point of hoping that the cancer confines itself to stage two not to save her son, but simply so that she doesn't have to despise another human being so completely. So that she doesn't have to shame the pediatrician by telling her she was wrong. So that she doesn't have to wound her by pointing out her incompetence. Lise feels, fleetingly, sorry for the woman. She doesn't understand that the ins and outs of her resentment are the only things helping her cope with this terrifying wait to hear the worst. A second thread now joins the first and complicates the woven pattern. It takes Lise back nearly a year to February 2012. Solal had been exhausted for two months and often went to bed when he came home from school. His skin, which was usually a healthy tan, had browned, gone almost greenish, and his eyes were hollow and deep set. He coughed a lot and didn't eat or sleep well. It was all the more surprising because he was basically never sick and went to the doctor only for vaccinations. But Lise had taken him to the pediatrician three times already since that January without securing any explanation or treatment. Smiley as ever, her son put on a brave

face for the doctor, who listened dubiously to their descriptions.
A clinical examination contradicted what they were saying. As
far as she could see, there were no grounds to take the matter
any further. Tired of this struggle, Lise eventually contacted a
GP as an emergency and asked for a full set of tests. It turned
out that Solal had just been through a period of glandular fever,
complicated by cytomegalovirus and pneumopathy. It took him
months to recover and he didn't look himself or regain his usual
vitality until the beginning of the fall. Just a few weeks, that is,
before the onset of the lymphoma. This more distant memory
revives the pain of the first by adding another color to it. Guilt
mingles in with the resentment. Why, Lise wonders, after this
first proof of incompetence, did I keep seeing that pediatrician?
Why did I have more faith in her questionable diagnoses than
my maternal intuition? Why did I submit to another person's
absurd obstinacy like that when I felt I was right? If those two
lost weeks mean the cancer has progressed to stage three, if Solal
needs a bone marrow transplant, if his chances of survival are
halved, if he dies, then, she tells herself, at the end of the day I'll
be responsible. Hating herself is definitely less difficult for Lise
to bear than hating someone else. It's high time the phone rang.

"Hello, it's me," says Olivier. I hold my breath. I don't know
what to say. I wait. "I just bumped into the nurse, they have
the results." Then there's a silence, probably only a short one

but it feels so long. I can't seem to break it. I wait again. The answer comes of its own accord. "It's not in his cerebrospinal fluid. It's stage two." I exhale an inarticulate sound. A cry of joy full of tears. Then the two of us, your father and I, stay there hanging on the phone without a word. We savor this momentary pause, balancing freely, entirely convinced that we'll fall the right way. We hear each other's breathing, heavy with emotion. I just say, "Don't move, I'm coming over," and hang up. My relief morphs into happiness, my happiness into exultation. I explode with joy. With the sound and fury of it. As my mother looks on, I jump around in every direction, knock over a chair, tear whole pages out of the newspapers, then rip them, screw them up, crumple them. I roll them into balls and throw these at the windows, thrilled by the way they bounce. Crazy, I've gone crazy. Crazy with euphoria. Crazy with jubilation. Crazy with this surge of hope. I don't think I've ever been so happy. Of course, the months to come will be extremely hard. Of course, this cancer will have terrible consequences and, whatever happens, our lives will have been irretrievably ravaged. Of course, nothing will ever be the same again. Of course, there's also the fact that you could still die. But I now have the strength to ignore it. The worst has been dodged and on that basis I forge profound faith in the victory ahead. I shall force myself not to lose sight of it.

———

Lise doesn't remember that day at the hospital. What was it like being reunited with her son? How was he feeling? What was he told about the results announced that morning? What did they do together? She doesn't know. As if, just like the initial trauma, her relief has erased part of her memory, making the intervening three days a sort of plateau between two dark chasms. Try as she might to trawl through its deepest recesses, her brain implacably refuses to reveal these memories. So she is left with nothing but a hiatus between the shock and the countershock.

One recollection does eventually emerge from this oblivion: a change of venue is needed. Not that Solal is finally allowed home, that's still not on the agenda, but right at the end of the afternoon he needs to go to a specialist medical center in the Eleventh Arrondissement for a cardiac ultrasound scan. Why outside the Institute? Lise doesn't remember and isn't sure she ever knew. What she does know, though, is that it's to check the implantation of the port-a-cath and to ensure her son's heart is functioning well following that intervention. For the purposes of this scan, then, Solal is given a sort of leave. It may seem banal, but the trip is a sufficiently noteworthy event to trigger Lise's memory again. Perhaps this is because, having embarked on a bizarre odyssey, it gradually restores the mother's awareness of the drama playing out in their lives.

"Could you put the siren on?" I dare to ask. I can't believe it. I turn to you and wink, you're exhilarated. To be honest, I don't know which of us is the more excited to be driving across Paris running red lights. But surely this horrendous week warrants a minor transgression. That must be what the ambulance driver thinks, because he complies with a smile. At first I enjoy it more than you do: sitting next to the driver, I'm intoxicated by the speed as we slalom between vehicles. I have a taste of free adrenaline, of an inconsequential fear that allows me to forget the other fear, the real one. It's definitely not so funny for you: lying in the back of the ambulance and hooked up to your drip, you can't see the road. You're just getting the sounds. So I make a point of turning around regularly to comment on our progress and share the adventure with you. Now we're at a crossroads. The lights are red. We plow through. A sedan and two electric cars pull into the median to let us through. They almost run into each other. Oops, a cyclist, on the right. Only just missed him. A scooter on the left. Make way, serf, restrain your ridiculous contraption and salute the passing of Solal the Great and his retinue. After we cross the River Seine, the commentary becomes unequivocally epic and we wend our way like the Chosen One parting the seas. We have the advantage of favorable winds from the man of a thousand ruses. We accomplish wonders and achieve the impossible. We're on fire as we reach the place de la Bastille, storming across it and taking flight down the boulevard Beaumarchais. When we reach the medical center the race is won. You're full of laughter and I feel nauseous. Oh, how we giggled.

I'm not a stranger to the place. I've been here for a number of consultations with your brother. For two reasons: first, Nils has been observed here since birth because he has a heart murmur. His cardiologist is the very man who'll be seeing you today, and I'm delighted by this happy coincidence. We have complete faith in Dr. Izoard; he ably handles the combination of empathy and distance, humanity and rigor that makes an excellent doctor. He always seems to be in the right place, and this appropriateness alone is enough to reassure patients. Memories of my last visit here, however, are less agreeable and likely somewhat to tarnish my relative serenity. It was only a few weeks ago. Nils had been complaining of stomach pains for months and we regularly saw blood in his stools. After encouraging us to be patient, his pediatrician eventually decided to send us to this same center for a consultation with a gastroenterologist, a Dr. Caprette. After the clinical examination, the doctor alluded to Crohn's disease and referred Nils for a colonoscopy to confirm her diagnosis. An appointment was set for early January at Necker Hospital; with children, the procedure is carried out under general anesthetic and they are hospitalized the evening before. I have to admit that the prospect of this, which naturally worried me at the time, has completely slipped my mind in the last few days. It's only when I heard our destination this afternoon that I remembered it, though as a secondary issue relative to the immediate emergency we were facing. But because fate is by its very nature mischievous, a series of minor incidents then starts, culminating in an inevitable pileup of all my misfortunes.

We're a motley crew entering the medical center that day. You walk in front, followed closely by a nurse holding in one hand the gray pump unit for your drip with a tube leading out of it that slips inside your coat, and in the other hand a green pouch connected to the pump. A second tube sets off from you and ends up, in my hands, at another pouch, this one filled with transparent fluid and also connected to the pump. We try our best to jog along at the same speed. In fact, all it takes is a change of pace—a momentary distraction, a hesitation about which way to go, or simply a step to the side—for the whole assemblage to be desynchronized. Sometimes it's a slowing: then we run into each other and scramble the tubes, the nurse steps on your heels, my face squishes into your back, and you come close to falling over. At others it's an acceleration that threatens our stability, and that's more serious. We risk breaking up. The pipes, being elastic, stretch, but they do eventually reach their limits. You give a little cry—the needle inserted into your port-a-cath moves and scratches you. If it tore out it would be a disaster. The liquid would spill over your skin, burning it with powerful active ingredients. So we advance cautiously, particularly as there are plenty of pitfalls. First we need to get through the heavy front door, then climb a few steps to the elevator, shuffle into the cabin, which is obviously too small to take the three of us, come out onto the landing on the third floor, go through the narrow doorway to the consultation center, and stand in line, the three of us in a row, at the reception desk. There are other parents in front of me, lucky parents holding their children by the hand. I can feel people looking at us. I understand; we do look kind of funny. Still, that's probably not why they let us go first. Either way, I'm grateful. Our trio goes by a single name and I announce it to the secretary: Solal M. The good-natured but narrow-minded computer finds an M. and proudly brandishes your brother, Nils. Just in case I'd forgotten him. The secretary hesitates, then perfectly logically looks for another appointment with Dr. Caprette. I correct her. "No, we're here to see Dr. Izoard." "Oh, yes, I'm sorry," the secretary says, still loyal to her machine, "your son also sees a cardiologist, I didn't look far enough back." "No, this is my other son, Solal, who's never seen either of these doctors." The secretary asks us the customary questions, then tells us to wait in the nearby room, Dr. Izoard is running a little late.

After some ten minutes you show signs of needing the bathroom. This is not as simple as it may seem. Since the

PET scan yesterday we actually have to collect your urine so that the amount of radioactive product evacuated can be calculated. Even though the substance is harmless, we have been asked to harvest the fluid in a large sealed receptacle, using latex gloves. This operation naturally acquires particular charm when performed outside the Curie. It's quite an adventure. First, we need to procure the accessories. The center's secretary may have no trouble finding disposable gloves, but she hits a snag on the container. Those available to her are either open or too small. Of course, I favor the closable ones because they will safeguard the fluid on its return to the Institute. Which is how I come to be in possession of four small sterilized plastic pots with red lids. As they are intended for scatology, they are identical to the pots that Dr. Caprette gave us to collect Nils's stools for analysis. Fully equipped, you make your way to the bathrooms, followed by the nurse and me still carrying our tubes, pouches, and pump. I squat at your feet, against the toilet bowl, using both hands to hold out a pot about four inches in diameter under your penis, which is distended by urinary pressure. The door to the stall stands wide open, and, thanks to the limited length of the tubes, the nurse has to stand in the doorway. You struggle to get the flow started. I can understand. The circumstances don't favor such intimacy. When your urine is finally released, things get complicated. The pot, being too small, is very soon full. I didn't anticipate this. I therefore have to interrupt you while I close the lid, put it to the ground, then grab a second pot, open its lid, and center it under the stream, which, despite your best efforts, is still flowing. I repeat this performance twice, gaining in dexterity and confidence with experience. We fall in step with each other's moves and find a rhythm. The handover goes with no losses for the next two pots. But as the volume of urine rises in the fourth, I realize that this last receptacle won't be enough to take it all. We've run out of pots. I need to fetch another. The situation is so outlandish that we burst out laughing, which incidentally isn't conducive to the necessary retention of your urine. I race out of the toilets, arriving disheveled in the waiting room, and skip the line of patients to ask the secretary—urgently—for more pots. By the time I return, the nurse has also succumbed to the comic absurdity of the scene. He roars as he tightens the last screw top. Mission accomplished, the three of us emerge from the toilets at our synchronized walk.

That is when we come across Dr. Caprette. She says hello, bringing an abrupt halt to our little group, and asks whether I'm here with Nils. No, just some pouches of glucose and chemo, a drip pump, some tubes, five pots of radioactive urine, a nurse, and my older son. I summarize the situation for her in a few words: lymphoma, last Monday, my other son, port-a-cath, cardiology. She offers to see me, after you've had your scan, to discuss Nils's problem. I agree without thinking about it, so long as you and the nurse are happy to wait before returning to the Institute. After this we don't stay long in the waiting room, but long enough to arouse curiosity. A few minutes later, Dr. Izoard comes for us. I'm happy to be reacquainted with this small, slight, and elegant man's sensitivity. As usual, he finds just the right thing to say, words that reassure while acknowledging pain and risk. We come out of the consultation calmer. Is it because of this feeling of confidence that I ask to see Dr. Caprette? Or because the secretary suggests it again when we pass her desk? Or simply because Nils has been mentioned so many times since we arrived here, gradually hammering away at me, reminding me that I really need to do it? In any event, I end up alone with Dr. Caprette in her office. We replay the conversation we had several weeks earlier, exploring your brother's intestines, the appearance, density, and frequency of his stools, the nature, origin, and duration of his pain, and the color, context, and volume of his bleeding. The same symptoms, the same causes, and the same effects as before. That *was* before, though. Everything is so different now. I find myself forced to postpone Nils's colonoscopy. Dr. Caprette doesn't understand, saying this problem needs dealing with as soon as possible. I'm surprised by her reaction and try to get her to say how serious Nils's condition is. It makes sense, I would think, to rank the emergencies. Her answer isn't clear, and feels more like a diatribe than a diagnosis, insidiously intermixing moral obligation with medical risks. I bring the conversation back to concrete facts. If this is Crohn's disease, couldn't we assume, given that the symptoms have remained mild for some period, that it is in an early or at least not very active phase? So aren't there other, less invasive tests that could be run first? I explain, again: given the family situation, I'm not in a position to have a second child hospitalized, even for one night, without a really serious reason. Besides, it strikes me as psychologically problematic to burden Nils with a night in the hospital and a general anesthetic, not to mention the especially intrusive nature of the colonoscopy itself, precisely when his brother's cancer is already presenting him with a medical situation that is particularly unintelligible for a child his age. So, unless there is immediate danger, I would prefer to wait a few weeks, to give the family time to rebuild some semblance of normality around this lymphoma. The gastroenterologist doesn't see it like that. As if, by prioritizing your oncological treatment, I've unwittingly attacked the importance she confers on her own specialty. Perhaps in doing this I've even devalued her personally. Her verbal diarrhea starts up again and swings toward invective. Dr. Caprette really needs to cure this incontinence, a stream of extremely insalubrious material. I try one last request, making it as basic as I can to avoid all possible ethical extrapolations: "In the worst-case scenario, if it deteriorates, are there non-surgical treatments?" In its simplicity, my question manages to staunch the verbal tide. "Yes, there's a whole battery of treatments for acute attacks: anti-inflammatories, immunosuppressants, corticosteroids." "Orally?" My obsession with tubes rears its head at last—it has to be said, the circumstances are ripe for it. For Nils, I want no intestinal probing, no oxygen mask, and no drip. "Yes, orally." "Well, then," I say, "that's fine. Let's postpone the examination till next month." This time Dr. Caprette is genuinely angry. She looks me up and down and then, exasperated, snaps, "You clearly don't understand. It's not cancer but it *is* serious. It's a disease I wouldn't wish on anyone. You should deal with it right away. If he hemorrhages it will be catastrophic." I resist her onslaught one last time: "Yes, but, as you said, it's not cancer. And for now it's manageable. We need to prioritize our problems, so I'll discuss this with my husband and call you. Thank you, Doctor."

Saturday, December 22. Day Six.

"Mrs. M? This is the Curie Institute. We're very sorry to have to inform you by telephone but we've just had Nils's results. They're not good. He has a tumor on the brain. It's an extreme oncological emergency. He needs hospitalizing for diode treatment this evening." Lise feels her body collapse. It's not designed to cope with this much. She can't have two sons undergoing chemo at the same time. She just can't. Anyway, come to think of it, it doesn't make any sense. How could a benign

127

intestinal illness deteriorate into cerebral cancer? No one, not even Dr. Caprette, ever mentioned this possibility. Lise doesn't understand at all. She tries, though. Rewinds through events. Which results are they talking about? To identify a tumor, they would need to have run tests on Nils. She doesn't remember a biopsy or a scan. Perhaps her memory is letting her down. Again. She searches, probes, but finds total darkness. She persists through the shadows. Tired of this fight, she eventually gives up on her stubborn mind. For a fresh start, better to concentrate on the body. Hers feels stiff and heavy. She swallows but her saliva gets stuck in her throat. She wiggles her fingers and toes. A shiver runs through her, stretching her skin and making the hairs stand up all the way down her back. Something bangs inside her head, a pulse growing stronger. "Diode, diode, diode, diode," it repeats obsessively. As it intensifies, the syllables disintegrate, their inflexion alters. "Oh die, oh die, oh die, oh die." Lise sits bolt upright in bed, eyes wide open. Her mind screaming in the silence.

Waking does nothing to dispel the terror. The turmoil of her dream explains it but this offers no relief. Reality and fantasy are inextricably intermingled; once again Lise understands their permeability. Once again, like on that first morning, but the other way around this time. Her discovery five days ago that you can live a nightmare means she can't banish this as a bad dream today. Regardless of common sense, regardless of logic. It's not rational, it's physical. Even though she knows Nils is unharmed, she needs a few hours to *feel it. Her very flesh struggles to accept it. She's needled by this dizzying unease for part of the morning. It clings to her skin and she can't shake it off. Nothing she does, no decision she makes escapes the shadow cast by her nocturnal fears. She must simply wait for its density to disperse and for the day to wear on. Its contours gradually slacken, the impression it left fades, the world becomes clearer. Reality reclaims its rights.*

With lucidity comes the strength to resist. Around noon Lise understands the violence from which the forcefulness and potency of her nightmare stemmed. The dream wasn't simply a desperate expression of the cruel coincidence that forced a mother to confront her two sons' different pathologies on the same day. It wasn't even a result of repeated crises. No, her agony dates from further back. And the dream revealed the forced intrusion of an opponent Lise has absolutely no time for at the moment: guilt. The news, at the beginning of the week, that Solal has cancer meant that daily life had to be reorganized around this disaster. A sort of realpolitik came into force and Lise felt that its self-evident logic was, if not a gift, at least an asset. Solal's illness had naturally redefined priorities, given decisions a pecking order, and resolved the question of what options were available. In this context, Dr. Caprette's insistence on rethinking the newly established order constituted an intolerable and destructive intrusion. She used the word "preference" for what was a necessity, and "choice" for what was an obligation. By comparing the two illnesses, by denying the perfectly exceptional nature of lymphoma, she

confronted the mother with an untenable dilemma. As if Solal's
life could not be saved without threatening his brother's. Now
back to her senses, Lise refuses to have this battle. She casts
around for the stand-in who can, on her behalf, ask for a sec-
ond opinion, gauge the scale of the danger, and explore other
solutions. She finds someone in the family: Mathilde accepts
the job and acquits herself of it with aplomb. An unhoped-for
gift: having a sister.

Tomorrow you'll be home. They gave us the news when we
arrived this morning. Tomorrow you'll be home.

How slowly this sixth and last day of your first spell in
the hospital is going. With your backaches and headaches.
With your first signs of nausea. With the smell of disinfectant, the torpor in the air, and the sound of machines. It
goes so slowly that I don't remember it. I'm left with almost
nothing of it. I'm left with just the music.

In fact, that very Saturday music comes back into our
lives at last. It has been setting the pace of our weekends
for more than a year. You and your sister on the piano,
me composing and singing. I've always known music was
there. I've always had a piano near me. A discreet presence,
a latent wish. But everything changed a few months ago:
when you started having your first lessons, your teacher
encouraged me to write, compose, and perform. I drew on

his experience for the legitimacy I lacked, and finally dared to do it. And I haven't stopped since. I can't put into words what it means to me. Perhaps it should be left in silence, and yet there's no denying our family life has been transformed. Music has insinuated itself into everything. It has expanded our space and extended our time. And now our home is constantly abuzz. It fills and empties with sounds and rhythms. As if it were breathing.

All of a sudden last Monday that breathing was interrupted. And now, five days later, music comes to the Institute. It's your teacher, Simon, who brings it back by agreeing to give you your weekly lesson. As if we were at home. As if nothing has changed. As if. A respect for habit is a pretense of normality and erases the oddness of the situation. Here in the middle of the corridor we take turns playing the piano. Then I'm brave enough to sing. Trauma gets the better of reserve. The accumulated tension spills out in musical passages that blot out the wheeze of pumps, the chatter of children, and the roaring silences. They bounce off the drab walls and tear through the stifled air. I'm worried about disturbing people, but the nurses tell me to keep going and soon people stop and listen: sick children, parents, caregivers. An audience gathers. A motley, eclectic group. The most indulgent listeners in the world. All they ask is to come along with you; they'd follow you anywhere, just so long as it's someplace else. Joy is a contagious thing; it spreads through the whole department and everyone joins

in: "If happy little bluebirds fly beyond the rainbow..."
There's still an if, though.

In the evening everything is calm again. Someone is
still whistling somewhere off down the corridor. A vestige
of the day. You're lying in bed trying to get to sleep. You
have a crisscross of tubes overhead for a dreamcatcher. You
open your eyes for a moment as if woken by an unresolved
thought. "You know the lead house, Mommy, the one we
talked about the other day? It happened. I think it's already
made of feathers." Your smile is so luminous, I wish I could
bottle it. I take you in my arms, my darling child, and sing
softly in your ear as you fall asleep. I know your house
won't be made of feathers for long. I know that soon the
whole protocol will crush your frail body. But I don't tell
you that. I let you escape into your fleeting dreams.

Tomorrow you'll be home.

7

There is one night and there is one morning, and then Solal is home. For three full days he is out of the hospital with his family. For three full days he is back among the healthy. Three days, from December 23 to 25. A long, restful Sunday rises over the new order. At first the idea seems such a happy one to the parents. They're being given back their son. They'll be able to reconstitute their family unit, that little domestic paradise in which each individual unsuspectingly savors the pleasure of being together. They've been told often enough: they must make the most of this, hugging each other close and celebrating their newfound togetherness around the Holy Child. In all honesty, they've been told it so often that it's become suspect. As if you must compulsorily be happy on December 24, when you're unhappy on the 23rd and could be in despair on the 25th. And yet it's clearly because of the date that this leave has been granted. It's the Christmas truce. Curie, 2012. Ypres, 1914. Should they be singing "Silent Night" amid the bombing, planting Christmas trees along the trenches, lighting candles on the front-line parapets, and exchanging gifts with the enemy on the front? Do they think the lymphoma is prepared to fraternize? It certainly would be wonderful if it rebelled against its fatal authorities. In the name of December 24, it could hold back its troops and slow the proliferation of malignant cells. And why not a remission to mark the occasion? The parents are clearly expected to park their anxieties, so the villain could lay down its arms. Unlikely, though. It's not that sort of humanist.

In return, Lise and Olivier are not inclined to make a pact. Even under normal circumstances they have an ambivalent relationship with this time of year. They loathe its culinary debauchery, its commercial pressures, and its spirit of hypocrisy, although they still enjoy the pleasures of the holiday season. Being anti-capitalists, they give lasting, ethical, and modest presents while surreptitiously coveting the technological feats acquired by a millionaire uncle. Being ecologists, they buy—at vast expense—a potted tree that, come January, will be driven in a diesel truck back to the forests of the Vosges region to be replanted. Being atheist and secular, they're touched by the fundamental symbol of a newborn lying in the hay, a fragile, helpless messiah. Being Bohemian and disenchanted, they poke fun at all the decorum and even privately fantasize about publicly outing some skeleton in the cupboard to breathe a bit of excitement into the atmosphere, but still every year they take turns visiting their families on

December 24 and New Year's Eve. Christmas is one of the rituals they deride while they can't actually do without it. But this year is different. Their hearts are not overflowing with joy. And in this context, any inducement to be happy feels almost like an ultimatum. Why make more of this Christmas Eve than usual? Won't there be others? Making something special of it would paradoxically constitute a sort of abdication in their confrontation with cancer. An unacceptable capitulation to the idea that this Christmas could be the last. This is probably why they accept and are not even offended by the fact that not one member of their respective families, apart from Lise's parents, joins them in Paris this year. After all, they've known for a long time that if they don't make the trip, the others won't come to them. What matters to Lise and Olivier is to give their children their usual modest Christmas. No more and no less.

Not much remains of these three days. Little nothings that add up to a lot. Simple pleasures. Affectionate gestures. And a constant swinging between the customary and the strange, a rocking that secretly soothes the household. First they decorate the tree. The same box brought up from the cellar, the same garlands, the same colors, the same lights, the same squabbles and laughter as the year before. But there's no argument this time that Solal should have the honor of putting the star at the top of the tree. Anna and Nils conferred and reached this decision. On their own. Their parents struggle to disguise their emotion. Olivier puts Solal on his shoulders and hoists him to the top. Lise puts her arms around the younger two. The ghost of The Last Christmas sidles through the evening air.

The next day, December 24, parents, children, and grandparents go for a walk in the Tuileries Gardens. It's a damp, gray day. The low, gloomy sky weighs on them uncomfortably. It's one of those winter days when life seems to be hampered. Even the cold isn't particularly apparent. The three children run ahead, raising dust on the path. They're wearing bobble hats, one navy blue, one gray, and one white, that disappear and reappear successively between the lifeless trees. As if withdrawing from the blandness of the day, only to pop out again a few yards farther on. Lise can't see or hear anything but her children. Everything else is just shadows and desolation. Their games, their chases, their cries, and their laughter reverberate in the silence. There is a sort of stridence to them that cuts right through her heart. Her very life howling on the edge of the precipice. Then all seven of them sit at a café table in the middle of the gardens. In among other people. Time stands still. The kids drink hot chocolate and the adults avoid eye contact. Solal is pale and tired. They need to go home now.

No one remembers the evening of the 24th, Christmas Eve. No more than they do the presents opened on the morning of the 25th. All that remains are a few words uttered by the youngest child over lunch. The three children are happy and noisy, having fun doing something they've been doing a lot the last few weeks, parodying a popular cartoon in which ghosts greet each other and announce wittily: "You look alive."

Nils studies his brother in silence, launches innocently into the familiar refrain, and then suddenly stops in mid-flow. "You look..." The words hang in the air—one second, an eternity—before plumping for a different adjective: "...immortal." So much for the ghost.

After lunch Solal sits at the piano in front of the whole family. A Chopin nocturne. His grandmother stands up, takes a picture, moves, takes another, changes angle, takes yet another, then another. It seems she can't stop capturing the moment. Who can blame her? And yet there's something tragic about this compulsive picture-taking. It's overwhelming. Her right eye masked by the device, her left—blinking in time with the photos—fills with increasingly visible tears. The ghost takes a seat and makes itself at home. Lise wishes her mother would stop. It's too painful. So she teases, makes fun, trivializes it to drive away the ghost. To be sure no one founders. On her invitation, they all take turns singing, miming, reciting a poem, or telling a funny story. Only this refusal to make an exception spares them from tragedy.

It's the afternoon already. You're lying on your bed. You've been in terrible pain for three days, in your back and head. To afford you some relief you have a white cotton headband around your forehead the whole time, and I regularly douse it with cool water. It makes you look like a Samurai, but you're very weak. You suddenly grab your comforter and roll it around you. I can't see your face now. You completely disappear under drifts of fabric. You stop moving. Stop talking. You've erased all trace of yourself. All that's left is this silent, motionless, shapeless mass. Then you peep your head back out slowly, still holding the comforter tight around your shoulders. Your face looks tiny against this huge body. Your headband has slipped halfway down over one eye. A frail pirate, gazing at me lovingly. You bury yourself under the fabric again and whisper in a tiny babyish voice: "Bye-bye, Mommy. I'm going back into my chrysalis and I won't come out for six months so I can fly away like a butterfly." What sort of flight do you mean? What are you flying away from? And where would you head? I don't know and maybe you don't either. What I do know, though, is that it's time to get you back to the Institute.

The truce is over. The hostilities begin again.

Exodus

PRESENT

No one just arrives at the hospital's inpatient wards; instead they really move in. This is because time works in its own unique way at the Institute. It has no past or future in the accepted sense of the terms. The past has been irrevocably abolished, and people survive here only at the cost of renouncing it. This tactic alone will sidestep regrets and remorse, the agonizing litany of ifs. The future has no citizenship rights either. People avoid thinking about it, shy away from hopes and plans. Tomorrow is another day, and no one really feels like contemplating it. And yet neither life before nor life after is truly eradicated. They simply belong to a different temporal dimension, and everyone understands that this dimension continues autonomously, in parallel. There is, however, a sort of tacit agreement between the department's different occupants that it is not acceptable to raise the subject. The outside world continues to beat out the rhythm of the seasons, working hours, school holidays, evening outings, and weekends in the countryside, while the micro-society at the Institute looks only to itself for support. In terms of normal chronology, then, the patient and his or her family live in *an eternal present. Which has its advantages. It produces a sort of reassuring routine. Here they can escape the weight of memories, the torments of decision-making, and the tyranny of time constraints. No one wonders what they should have done or should do next. A superior order now governs every initiative. They're not resigned to it; they collaborate with it. Uniformity prevails. Each day follows the last, all of them alike. Patients wake, bathe, eat, find diversions, and nap at the same time. The same stifling temperature holds sway summer and winter. Enveloping everyone and sending them to sleep. Shutters lowered, curtains drawn, neon bulbs produce a dull monotonous light night and day. Everyone consents graciously to this pretense of permanence. Everyone kills time in his or her own way. The children, when they're well enough, go to the playroom, the art room, or the schoolroom, they read comics, watch TV, and—mostly—sleep. Their parents comfort, wash, tend, feed, and kiss them, then, when their child is asleep or in the care of the staff, try to find distractions: also the TV, and comics too, coffee, cigarettes, the piano . . . Most of them readily adapt to the local customs. They've taken up residence at the Institute and sink unresisting into its torpor. They brought their slippers, their pajamas, their favorite pillows, and they wander the corridors in their nightwear until the middle of the day.*

And yet this regressive comfort is delusional. It cannot exist without an abdication of freedom. Subject to the diktats of treatment, enslaved by endless repetitions of prescribed gestures, the citizens of the Curie devote themselves to a single task—waiting—while another merciless timescale plays out in secret. Cancer reigns supreme, decreeing its own rhythm and prescribing its chronological units. Treatment protocols stand in for years, chemotherapy sessions for months, periods of aplasia and infections for weeks, lumbar punctures, bouts of mucositis, and drip-fed meals for days. Pouches of drugs are replaced on drips hour after hour. Nausea and pain come in successive waves minute after minute, while the wheeze of drip pumps counts out the seconds. Monotony, just like eternity, is only an illusion. Its tempo is irregular. Its routines still harbor emergencies. All at once and with no warning, everything accelerates. Sudden vomiting, a sharper pain, the alarm on a pump, vital-signs monitors galloping—all things that mean a nurse must be called urgently or someone must even run to fetch help. Any hurrying disrupts the department's steady purr and brings concern for the future back into sharp focus. Then there's no point pretending. And the pulse of time can be heard again. "Remember," it says, "it's five chemo sessions, four aplasias, and sixteen lumbar punctures, in other words exactly a quarter to remission." Enough to make you scrap your slippers.

As is always the case with temporal telescoping, whenever outside-world time meets Institute time, a sort of paradox occurs. But definitely not in the way science fiction interprets the word. In fact, it's impossible to travel to the past here. The past can be regretted, but at the Institute there's no possibility *of altering the chain of causality. The cause of a cancer can neither be eliminated from the past, nor the chances of the patient's recovery be improved in the future. No one ever travels back. Besides, this paradox isn't due to a series of contradictory facts; instead it insinuates itself into people's words and reactions. Into their ambivalence. It therefore borders on the absurd, and leaves an uncomfortable feeling. Lise has a painful experience of this one day with Jeanne, the mother of seven-year-old Marion. In the course of conversation, Jeanne confides to Lise that her daughter's nephroblastoma has now spread to her lungs and the metastasized tumors are stage four. She's been told they're terminal. In trying to relieve the child's suffering and do the best for her, the oncologists are hesitating between palliative chemotherapy and surgery involving curettage of the metastasized areas. Jeanne is hesitating too. For different reasons. The problem is, she says, although she dreads the side effects of one final course of chemotherapy, she's worried the surgical intervention would leave very visible scars on her daughter's chest. She wouldn't want these to be a hindrance to Marion's life as a woman when she grows up. And that's the crash. The terrifying pileup of realities. Here, there's a little girl dying. There, she has a future. Here, she will always be seven years old with a child's body, narrow hips, and a flat chest. There, her womanhood blossoms, she has relationships, lovers, maybe children. Here, the end. There, tomorrows. "What would you choose?" Jeanne asks Lise, "chemo or surgery?" "I don't know," Lise replies, appalled. "Have you* asked your daughter?" Lise is lying. In actual fact she knows exactly what she'd choose. She'd choose to rewind the clocks so that she never had to deal with this conversation.

Cases of temporal paradox like this are, thank goodness, rare. Everyone makes a point of avoiding them. And there is a solution to achieving this. It consists in losing oneself in the moment. Investing in the Institute's day-to-day life, succumbing to its laws, conforming to its customs, surrendering to its rituals. Concentrating on what needs doing and, when there's nothing left to do, watching the surrounding microcosm, contemplating it even. Studied for long enough, every gesture, every individual, every object can diffract into a multitude of elements, affording the eye and the mind endless subdivisions of possibility. And this rekindles a semblance of curiosity and amazement. A form of poetry protects the watcher from the unthinkable. And the here and now survives thanks to the voice of things.

STIRRER

It's one of those afternoons when nothing's happening.
Which should be a good sign: it presupposes that no
aggressive medical intervention is scheduled, that you
don't have a fever, you're not in pain, you're vomiting less,
and you may be asleep. So I have nothing to do. I'm waiting for you to wake. Waiting till you need me again. In-
activity does entail its share of risk, though. I mustn't use
this opportunity to start thinking. There's no way I could
cope with the consequences. Here I am, then, killing time
to avoid boredom. Unable to fall asleep in the armchair in
your room despite being tired, I decide to procure myself
some energy from the vending machine in the cafeteria on
the second floor. I usually have a cup of tea and a chocolate bar. It's not such a brilliant idea. Although officially
intended as somewhere that patients and their visitors can
relax, the cafeteria is probably the grimmest place in the
hospital. As depressing as can be. This isn't due only to
the insipid lighting that filters through the metal slats over
the perennial neon lights. Nor even the convulsive and
completely maddening way one of them blinks. In fact, a

whole raft of factors seems to have been combined here to transform a break into an ordeal. For a start, the room's proportions don't feel appropriate. While the staff on the sixth floor constantly struggle with a lack of space, competing in their inventiveness to accommodate treatment rooms, playrooms, administrative offices, and extra bedrooms, the cafeteria four floors down occupies a good three hundred square feet with impunity. This wouldn't be so scandalous if the place were inhabited, but most of the time the tables sit empty. Vending machines dispense drinks and food to the few occasional visitors, who are mostly in a hurry to consume them somewhere else. No one wants to stick around. The place feels desperately lifeless. Everything about it is inert. Efforts have clearly been made to introduce some sort of decoration to cheer the space up. A trellised arbor in varnished wood, a few potted plants, timidly suggesting an indoor garden. Except that these plants aren't breathing. They're artificial. A fake creeper lolls lazily along the far wall. Its artlessly imitated stem forks into a series of covered metal branches, each of which divides again into dozens of secondary offshoots, and these in turn split with mechanical regularity into batches of three nylon leaves. It's doubly miserable because it's ugly.

At least I don't have to fight for a free seat. I have too much choice; the place is empty. I sit at the table in the middle, equidistant from the creeper and the entrance, filling the space as best I can. Now I need to fill my time. I explore the accessories at my disposal. First a Kit Kat, in other words four wafer biscuits covered in milk chocolate. This can be made into a routine, which is a good thing. Tearing the paper, snapping off a finger of biscuit, eating it slowly, taking another, looking at the strata of wafer, caramel, and chocolate, eating them all together, then repeating the performance. On the fourth finger I feel sick. It's full of sugar, palm oil, cheap cocoa, and artificial flavorings. And, what's worse, it's used up barely five minutes. The tea is scarcely more satisfying. Soaking in inadequately heated water, a teabag full of torn, shredded, and crushed black leaves dispenses a beverage that manages to be both weak and bitter. I make the displeasure of it last as long as I can, and painstakingly gain another five minutes. This afternoon is definitely dragging its heels. I'm suddenly tired, and this comes coupled with attendant anxiety and gloominess. With the Kit Kat finished and the teacup drained, I think I've exhausted my resources. But I'm wrong.

Without thinking, I pick up the stirrer that the vending machine supplies for hot drinks. This disposable object is about four inches long. Usually plastic but sometimes wooden, they can come in several different shapes, depending on whether the spatula aspect of it appears at the end of a handle or all along its length. It might also include some whimsical details, mainly cutouts that may be circular, semicircular, oval, or diagonal, and in groups of three, four, or five, allowing free circulation of the drink to help stir it.

In fact, if you can forget the crass material, its modest size, and the mediocrity of its use, it can look like an antenna on an innovative piece of technology, a lacy hair accessory, a peculiar kind of key, or a mysterious symbol. To be honest, the one I have possession of this afternoon doesn't give the imagination much purchase. It's a standard model in white plastic, flat in shape and uniform in width. It has no grooves or apertures. It's apparently destined to create only mild turbulence. And yet I'm still intrigued by it. Interest born of boredom, some would say.

First, I amuse myself considering its name. Not "mocha spoon," "beverage blender," or just "spatula." Oh no. These things have a word to themselves. And that is "stirrer." It may not be a particularly elegant word but there's a sensuous gentleness to its assonance—stirrer, stir, fur, purr, pearl, whorl, curl, unfurl—that conjures poetic images of the natural world. It also has a subtle energy that grows progressively in an irresistible, ever-increasing vortex from a slender implement to blend the ingredients of my canteen tea all the way to the childhood thrills of a dizzying fairground ride via an eddying kaleidoscope of associated words and sounds... stirrer, stirring, whirring, churning, turning, twisting, shifting, swirling, whirling, whirling dervish, whirligig, topsy-turvy, hurly-burly, higgledy-piggledy, helter-skelter. Good. Time is passing at last.

As I pursue my reveries, I instinctively put the stirrer on the edge of the table. While my left index finger holds

a good third of its length firmly on the Formica, my right
index flicks its remaining length that sticks out over thin
air like a diving board. As I strike it, the stirrer starts to
vibrate up and down, giving off a muted hum. Visually, it's
magical. It looks as if the unsecured portion of the thing is
defying the laws of physics. Usually rigid, it becomes flex-
ible, almost elastic. This is because, racing to stay abreast
of the rapidly alternating image, my brain struggles to keep
the messages up-to-date. If I further accelerate the movement, it even gives the impression of a continuum. As if
the object has become so rubbery that it stretches out vertically like kneaded dough before resuming its normally
rigid form. This phenomenon soon proves hypnotic and the
need to repeat it obsessive. I feel as if I could spend hours
watching the effects produced by my finger like this. But
another sensation short-circuits the experiment, giving it
an auditory dimension that eventually turns out to be far
more rewarding and fruitful. The stirrer's vibrations are accompanied by a characteristic sound. Every flick administered to the thing—augmented in a series of knocks against
the table—sends out waves that make the particles in the
air oscillate for a few seconds. So that I experience a sort of
second-degree vibration: I hear what I see. It's not long before I identify a degree of musicality in it. Of course, its tim-
bre is not especially subtle. But it *is* unusual. Interestingly,
the stirrer doesn't produce perfect notes. The frequencies
are too approximative to emit the pure sound of a tuning

fork or the complex sound of a real musical instrument. It's difficult to reach high notes to fit perfectly into a scale, and yet I have a strong sense that the stirrer's every vibration is a fundamental frequency and a sort of harmonic. In fact, it all depends on the sine curve of the sound, which is faithfully proportional to the amplitude of the stirrer's movement. The longer the section undergoing these oscillations, the larger the acoustic curve and the deeper the note. The shorter I make the free part of the stirrer, the higher up the scale we go. While there's no guarantee of hitting exact notes, then, it is at least possible to ensure clear and regular intervals between the sounds. Lastly, the duration of these vibrations allows for different rhythms, while their intensity opens up the possibility of varying dynamics. It's fascinating. Here in this desolate place, somewhere between an artificial plant and a coffee dispenser, a piece of plastic comes to life and becomes a means of making music.

As I explore how to put this to best use, I first take pleasure in considering the overall shape of the sound. I savor its evolution: its initial attack, the sustained note, its diminuendo and eventual extinction. What I really want is to follow each emission to the very end, to lose no part of what is physically audible, to spoil no element of each musical exhalation. I sometimes need to close my eyes to help me hear its decline. The time eventually comes to play the instrument, and I soon identify two different techniques. The first consists in moving the stirrer backward and forward over the edge of the table during a single set of vibrations. By striking the thing firmly and sharply, the sound produced can last sufficiently long for me to modify it at leisure. This method produces rising and falling chromatic sequences. Conversely, the second technique involves applying a series of staccato flicks while modifying the instrument's alignment with the edge of the table each time. With repeated experimentation it's then possible to identify the ideal position to produce a particular note. It might even be worth graduating the stirrer, like the frets on a guitar, in order to return to each sound more easily. As I have neither a pencil nor something sharp enough to scratch the plastic, I default to using my sensory memory. With the help of increasing experience, I'm gradually able to locate the note I want with the first strike, and I then have fun clumsily reproducing a few famous nursery rhymes: "Au clair de la lune," "Frère Jacques," and "Ah! Vous dirai-je, maman." I pay particular attention to the last of these because of the multiple possibilities offered by Mozart's variations on the theme. So I linger over it. Gaining in confidence, I eventually get carried away and devise my own successions of sounds, although I wouldn't go so far as to describe them as melodies. By combining the two playing methods, I think it would be possible to produce, if not an infinite number, at least a huge variety of musical compositions. Due to the harmonic inaccuracy of the instrument, the most difficult thing is not creating a melody but reproducing it. I decide to explore this area and to attempt some progress here. I repeat and double-check each note dozens of times. More specifically, I anchor their position in a percussive rhythm by beating out time with my foot and index finger. I'm integrating the sounds in a time signature. This gives a distinctive character to each of my little creations. Then I syncopate and sigh, I play before and after the note, out of time. I also have fun varying the tempo. Largo, lento, adagio, moderato, allegro, presto. And then ad libitum. Institute time no longer matters. The minutes go by and I don't notice them. I have better things to do.

Someone does eventually come into the cafeteria. He's come to the wrong place, that's clear. He very soon leaves again, anyway. Still, it's enough to break my concentration. I look at the clock and realize I've been playing the stirrer for nearly two hours. I find this idea particularly charming, although faintly ridiculous. It really doesn't make any sense. Letting myself get so wrapped up in a simple piece of plastic. I think I've sunk very low, I can't have much left if it's come to this. Maybe just a tiny snippet. And a tiny snippet is a very good start. I also think you must be awake by now and you're going to laugh when you hear about my adventure. And that's a very good reason to go back to your bedside.

BEAN

I t's a piece of cardboard about eight inches long and
shaped like a bean. Or a kidney. Molded fibers ensure
its strength. Granted, it's not as durable as its plastic or
stainless-steel counterparts. It's for single use. Disposable.
But I can imagine it's biodegradable and recyclable. Its simple lines and neutral color lend it an austere quality associated with objects intended for salvaging. Perhaps it already
comes from other, former existences and is destined to endless
rebirths. There's something paradoxically reassuring about
picturing this trash eventually crushed, pulped, cleaned,
drained, pressed, and dried to begin a new life cycle. Despite
the symbolic hope offered by this palingenesis of waste, it
doesn't keep Lise's interest for long. No more than the botani-
cal or anatomical metaphors regarding its curves. At best, this
thing reminds her of the limbless little creature curled around
its neuronal tube that ultrasound scans reveal to future parents in the fourth week of pregnancy. Except that no heart
beats in the middle of this. It's an inert gray embryo, filled
with something that stinks, and the mother's sole aim is to
get rid of it as soon as possible. Period. Because it's here, into

the endlessly repeated avatars of this recipient, that her son throws up all day. It's also here that he keeps spitting. So its content is either more or less liquid, depending on the expelled substance. The color scheme varies too. Vomit, although directly connected to the last meal, has its favorite shades. It can produce a disparate palette from white through to dark brown with a predominance of yellows, oranges, and dark reds. Sometimes greige, tan, putty, pink, vermillion, scarlet, or carmine, sometimes amber, vanilla, corn, or saffron. Occasionally it veers to completely green, and then turns olive, chartreuse, sludge, or goose dropping. But most of the time it's very light, almost transparent. The child eats hardly anything. His stomach is empty. He has only bile, gastric juices, and mucus to offer. A sort of pure vomit, whose transparency is matched by its indeterminate olfactory qualities. It never smells of regurgitated pasta, meat, yogurt, or banana. It just smells of vomit. His spittle, on the other hand, has no pretensions to plurality. It's even disconcertingly monotonous. Virtually odorless, it also presents no polychromatic tendencies. It is invariably pale pink. The result of a combination of saliva and solutions designed to prevent oral infections. Because the child is subjected to regular mouthwashes, intended to fight off bouts of mucositis that flourish thanks to the effects of aplasia. To this end, he has a small plastic bottle with his name on it in which he mixes one part of Paroex to ten parts of water every morning. Then he takes a mouthful of the mixture five or six times a day, gargles it around his ulcers, and spits the

*whole lot out into the cardboard bean. Added to this voluntary
spitting, there are less-controlled excretions. The patient can
be gripped by truly compulsive salivation, and it isn't clear
whether this is due to the chemotherapy, the Paroex, or a nervous reaction. So the child moves about with a bean in his
hand at all times, or he balances one—ready for use—on the
handle of his drip pole. This space seems to have been designed
with the specific purpose of accommodating the thing: the bean
fits exactly into the area where a hand would usually be put
to push the pole, and its curved rim rests against the metallic
handle. The perfect match between these two quite separate
things affords the mother a sort of satisfaction that constantly
amazes her. Somewhere, in secret, some sort of order seems to
oversee everything.*

I walk discreetly along the corridor, holding your latest production at arm's length, as I take it to dispose of it in the
bedpan washer. I don't want to keep throwing it in the trash
can in the toilet adjoining your room, as I did in the early
weeks. I'd perfected a procedure: turning the bean over so
that the liquid flowed to the bottom of the plastic container
while the cardboard could act as a lid, then covering the
whole lot with a multitude of diverse trash—magazines,
newspapers, paper, half-eaten desserts, and used gloves.
But it had a persistent smell and, even with the door closed,

the smell always seeped into your room eventually. I don't want you living in that stench any longer, no more than I want to share it with your partner in misfortune in the other bed. I don't want to go on calling a nurse ten times a day so she in turn can hound a cleaner to empty the trash regularly. A pointless waste of time and energy for everyone. So I've adopted the bedpan washer solution. Tucked away in a tiny space opposite the nurses' room, the device is designed to empty, rinse, and disinfect bedpans, urinals, commode chair buckets, diuresis containers, and other receptacles for human waste. I don't know why I've convinced myself it's not legitimate to empty the contents of the cardboard beans here, before putting the bean itself into the nearby trash. This qualm definitely doesn't relate to its shape: ergonomic, round, oblique, oblong, with handles, spouts, stoppers, covers, and adaptations; every kind of receptacle is accepted indiscriminately. My embarrassment must be down to the material and the single-use nature of these beans. If they were made of glass, plastic, or stainless steel, if they could be washed and sterilized, I would probably be less reluctant to empty the beans into the contraption. Unless I've subconsciously established a hierarchy of excreta. In that case, only waste from the lower half of the body—defecation and urine—would be admitted, while oral emissions—vomit and spit—would have no right to be here. I can't say. In any event, I'm certainly ashamed. Not only do I feel that I'm breaching a taboo by entering a room reserved for hospital staff, but I also have a sneaking sense of impropriety. In the same way that you yourself can't bear throwing up in front of anyone else, you also hate having the residue of your suffering exhibited like this. It means that some intimate part of yourself escapes the closed confines of your room. And I can understand that for you this is particularly obscene.

So I hug the walls, clutching the full bean in one hand while the other struggles to hide its contents. In vain. Even spread out, my hand is too small, barely covering half of the fluid. In any event, the smell gives us away. It's always with me, following me everywhere, sometimes preceding me. Most of the time I need travel only a few yards like this. And that's plenty. But sometimes your room is farther from the emptying site. My embarrassment is then bolstered by a technical challenge: ensuring, for the duration of the journey, that I don't spill anything. An incident would be the height of shame. A moment's distraction, a misstep, an overfull container, and disaster strikes: the liquid overflows, droplets escape, and a dribble darkens the linoleum in the corridor. If this happens I have no choice but to move faster, thereby renewing and increasing the risk of further spillages, so that I can get rid of the contents in the bedpan washer as soon as possible. Then, without wasting a minute, I must come back and ask a cleaner for a floor mop, all the while refusing her help with a no-thank-you-ma'am-you're-so-kind-I'll-do-it-myself. And it's tough luck for my discretion. Not to mention the time—only once—when I

don't see the small yellow couch opposite the door to where
the bedpan washer is. Even though it's always been there. I
know it well. I've even had occasion to sit on it. But on this
particular day, for some obscure reason—I'm distracted
or anxious, I bump into someone unexpectedly, or I come
across a child with a drip and give way to him—I stupidly
don't notice it. My right foot knocks into the base while my
left foot is already embarking on a large, decisive step. I'm
put off balance. I sway, topple, try to right myself. I have
only one free hand, and on top of that it's the less deft of
the two, and it beats the air desperately, trying to find purchase. The other hand automatically frees itself, hotly abandoning its load and stopping my fall, at the last moment, by
grasping the back of the sofa. Six feet away, the bean lies
pitifully on the floor, upside down amid an explosion of
vomit. It's everywhere. On the linoleum, the walls, the door
to the washer, and a nurses' cart. The smell is unbearable.
Members of the staff come running. They help me get to
my feet and clean up the corridor. I cooperate meekly, beyond shame. The incident even amuses me in the end and I
laugh out loud. After all, what does it matter. I succeeded.
The corridor may be spattered but the only smell in your
room is the bitter tang of sterilizing chemicals.

THE BEAN, ONCE AGAIN,
BUT MAGIC

L ong before Solal came to the Institute, beans already
fueled his imagination. Not the cardboard type, whose
prosaic medical purpose we now understand so well,
but the vegetal variety that has far more promising artistic
possibilities. It was when Solal was seven or eight. He wanted
to take musical theater classes, so his parents signed him up
for a weekly class at the local community center. The children
in the course were rehearsing for a show at the end of June, a
sort of pop-rock opera, a modern version of the popular "Jack
and the Beanstalk" story. The libretto, which was in verse,
featured a galaxy of eccentric characters and a quirky sense
of humor that harbored the occasional note of sadness. Lise
had bought the CD and the whole family knew all the songs by
heart. She and her children sometimes even acted out passages
on Wednesday afternoons, when there was no school, sharing
the roles and singing the chorus of the title song together. They
each had their pet song, but there was one on which they all
agreed; it was called "And So It Goes." It was sung by Jack's
mother, a sort of sugar-coated Mother Courage, and it prof-
fered a simple wisdom through rudimentary metaphors set to

a melancholy tune. It described the wheel of fortune turning through alternate showers and sunshine, sorrows and smiles, winters and summers, dark corridors and bustling life. The melody was just as modest as the lyrics, but the overall effect still proved touching, and perhaps even appealing for being so accessible. There was an aesthetic to its obviousness. In February that year the whole family had been to see an adaptation of the original opera in a small Paris theater. This musical fairy tale had therefore become a cultural reference for the family even before Solal delivered his performance in it.

The child had wanted to keep his part in the show a secret. Other members of the family had tried their best to get him to speak. To no avail. And so each of them came up with his or her own hypothesis: Nils saw Solal as the truculent ogre, Anna as a rock star cockerel surrounded by adoring hens, his father as the good and sensitive Jack, and his mother as the ironic virtuoso of a narrator. Naturally. When it came to the end-of-year production, amid the glories of the Fifth Arrondissement's Mairie on the place du Panthéon, they were in for a surprise. Solal was playing an unexpected part: kneeling, with his hands pressing down on the top of his head and his neck bent to one side, he represented the bag of beans. A character study, for sure, and one that must have been quite a challenge, starting with the need to stay silent and motionless for a whole hour. Still, his parents couldn't help feeling he was being underutilized, and some part of them cherished the hope that it would all come good in the second half. And Solal did indeed have a promotion: he now personified the magic beanstalk itself. This involved a good deal of choreography: the starting position was the same, but he then had to crouch down on his heels and, from there, rise slowly and, undulating all the while, point his joined hands toward the sky to mime the plant germinating and shooting up out of the bean. Then he spread his outstretched arms and opened his hands to form a tree-like shape, indicating that the beanstalk had reached the giant's castle in the clouds.

The family laughed about this anecdote for a long time. Solal was teased about his instinct for comedy, his subtle performance, and his vegetal inclinations. They also poked fun at the poor standard of the drama teaching offered by the course, deeming it a complete waste of time and money. Now, though, it seems the investment wasn't such a bad one. That musical fairy tale has in fact found a new use at the Institute, because these ubiquitous cardboard beans keep waking memories of that ebullient artistic fiasco. In the first instance, just remembering it is enough to amuse both mother and son, and then their memories take root and start to grow: the characters, the tunes, and the songs come back along with all that Wednesday-afternoon laughter. Each of them draws on his or her own experience at the time. It grows, spreads, and blossoms luxuriantly. They can still live well for having lived so happily. Soon they don't really remember but invent and devise from scratch. Every new cardboard bowl is welcomed by the musical's title song, and the mother accompanies it with a little extemporized dance. At first hesitant, this sequence is gradually perfected and eventually constitutes an established routine that the child gladly performs himself when he feels strong enough. With her elbows bent and hands at chest height, twirling the bean bowl in quick circles from left to right and then right to left, she beats out the rhythm by crossing and uncrossing her feet at the foot of the bed, producing a dance with a vague music hall feel to it. It's ridiculous and clumsy and has a hint of the Maurice Chevalier about it, with a scrap of cardboard standing in for a boater, a hospital room for the stage, and a sick child as the only audience. And yet it manages to transform the space. Every little performance is an interlude that unfailingly offers an opportunity for escape. With time, this diversion becomes a ritual and one type of bean systematically quashes the grimmer connotations of the other. It's reduced to fiction. By a sort of Pavlovian reflex, nausea produces anticipation for this entertainment. It wouldn't take much for vomiting to be synonymous with singing, dancing, and then laughing. Of course there's an element of tragedy in these moments. These happy reprises of the refrain are deceptive, and both Lise and Solal know they are. They can't help but remind mother and son of the true drama being played out here. And no one can be sure whether they are in fact secretly singing a quite different song. And so it goes, yes, maybe. But the ploy still works and sadness is dispelled for a few minutes. Perhaps at the end of the day the bean really is magic.

AN APARTMENT

The pediatrics department at the Institute is an apartment. It has its bedrooms and bathrooms, its dining room and kitchen, its playroom and balconies. In the Fifth Arrondissement it's a luxury. But it is shared. There are only eighteen beds and few single rooms. But each double room is a sort of suite with a wash basin and private toilets. One of them even has a full bathroom. It's not the loveliest of the rooms, though, because the window doesn't open. The only air anyone breathes there is inside air that's been circulated, evacuated, and reintroduced by the air-conditioning. All the rooms have names, rather like vacation cottages. It's better than a number. A name can fuel dreams or raise a smile, take people on a journey or remind them of childhood. The young patients change rooms with each new course of chemotherapy. Sometimes, though, they need to move during the course if they develop an infection. In these instances they're isolated so as not to infect the others. On the whims of chance and necessity, then, they find themselves assigned to Palm Trees, Pirouette, or Frangipani. It's a sort of musical chairs. When they get a single room, they're not keen to give it up, but are well aware that it will probably be occupied *by someone else next time. These places are temporary, but each individual inhabits and appropriates them in his or her own way: the child's name stuck to the door, photos held to a metal board with magnets, pictures Scotch-taped to the walls, words and hearts traced through the film of dust on the windows. Lise has made a large poster for her son, a patchwork of pictures, memories of holidays, and get-well cards, and she transports it from room to room to establish some continuity and familiarity after each change. This means Solal has a nomadic, movable home that spares him a feeling of transience.*

Children sleep with their parents in this apartment. Or rather with one parent; that's the rule. Each child must choose whether Mom or Dad will sleep in the cot set up next to his or her own bed. Which means that in the double rooms, there are four people sleeping—if, that is, they can get any sleep. Parents are tolerated, but don't really live in the apartment. They're viewed more as subletters or stowaways. During the day they must fold up their beds and tidy away their belongings so as not to hinder their child's treatments. Every trace of their nocturnal presence disappears. Travelers with no luggage. There are no showers for them either. The communal bathrooms are reserved for patients, and there are two of them: the little one and the big one. Solal prefers the larger one. Not that the difference in size is significant, but this one has recently been refurbished and has a hydraulic bathtub. A water pressure jack can be activated by remote control to alter the height of the bath. The purpose of this is clearly ergonomic: it's designed to make the tub more

accessible to patients with reduced mobility, and to their caregivers. Because children are bathed by their parents here, even
when they're young teenagers. This is down to the fact that it's
not easy taking a bath when you're connected by a tube to a
metal pole on wheels. First, you have to take off your clothes,
then step into the tub, sit down, and soap yourself, being careful
not to submerge the tube. It's easier for the parent to help the
child climb into the tub when it's in a low position, and then
activate the raising device to bring the tub up to adult standing
height while the child is washed. But Solal isn't especially interested in these technical considerations. What he likes is playing with the remote control, raising the bath as high as it will
go, on a level with his mother's head, then dropping it down as
quickly as the laboring hydraulic hoist will allow. This guarantees some explosive laughter and some accidents, which in turn
usually produce more laughter. So they have taken to securing
the chemo tube to the side of the resin tub with Scotch tape. But
if they don't think to leave any slack, then when the bath goes
up, the tape peels away and the tube drops into the water. They
retrieve it hastily, dry it, and check the needle is still inserted.
This usually causes a good flurry of panic. If, on the other hand,
the tension on the tube ends up pulling out the port-a-cath needle, it's a lot less amusing. A few drops of the drug escape, and
that's an emergency. This isn't to do with the momentary pause
in the treatment, nor a stringent need to measure how much
medication has been lost, nor even the cost of this waste, but the
risks associated with these substances coming in contact with

the skin. The affected area then needs to be rinsed copiously, dried, and disinfected. Lise has always wondered why such a fuss is always made over a single drop on the skin when Solal's internal tissues have to cope with several cups of the stuff every day. She has never had an answer to this question. In any event, bath time is normally a happy event that mother and son can share. One time, however, an uncle of Solal's who had come to visit helped him with his bath instead of Lise. Solal threw up in the water that day. As he had on previous occasions. It produced long orangey trails that distorted as they undulated on the surface, and fluffy clumps that sank slowly to the bottom of the tub. The uncle called for a nurse and a cleaner. And then he left, never to return. A child's privacy is a relative concept in this apartment.

The kitchen is next to the dining room and connected to it by a hatch. They're not large rooms; they don't really need to be. Not many people eat here, anyway. The patients can choose from a menu here, but few of them make use of this. The side effects of chemotherapy preclude normal eating habits. There are too many bouts of nausea and mucositis. But, driven by their curiosity, a fleeting improvement, or a parent, some do venture here. First they must brave the tepid salty canteen smell that turns their stomachs. Then they totter over to the single communal table and try to find a seat with enough space to park their drip. Plus, they need to locate an accessible socket to plug in the pump for fear of it bleeping. On their way to the table, children often get their feet or their drip tangled in the leads supplying *other pumps. It's a small space, after all. There are only about eight chairs. When there are too many people, any adults present make way for the patients. This doesn't happen much. The dining room is more often than not empty. Most of the children eat in their beds, if and when they're not being fed parenterally. Next comes the choice of food. The cook, a tiny slip of a woman who is both bossy and cheerful, announces the options through the hatch. She doesn't appear straightaway; only the sounds of her voice and her hands busying away in the kitchen carry through the opening. The children dither for a long time. They clearly don't really feel like any of it. Each dish named repels them a little more. At this point the cook leans on her elbows through the hatch. She negotiates, promises, and adapts to awaken their appetites. She excels at this tactic, slowly gaining territory, and can usually serve up a little something for each of them. Sadly, she enjoys only rare triumphs. Sickness very often wins hands down over hunger. It's not unusual for someone to throw up in the dining room of this apartment. No one comes close to being offended, not even the cook who has prepared food in vain, yet again. When the children have gone to bed, it's the adults' turn to eat at the communal table. They are not entitled to the Institute's menus—here too they are merely visitors. Instead, they must bring food in from outside, store it in the large shared fridge, and heat it up in the microwave. Which does nothing to help the smell. The parents often feel nauseous too. In their case, this is mostly down to overload, if not indigestion. Too much to think about, too much pain, too much worrying.*

And, truth be told, too much anarchic food as well. Because, in keeping with an equation peculiar to this apartment, the less the children eat, the more the parents snack. After they've had their own breakfast in the morning they pick at the bread left on the patient's tray. After lunch they polish off the rejected mashed potato, meat, and yogurt. Before having their own evening meal, they gulp down the neglected soup and Camembert without thinking. Not to mention the pastries, caramels, chocolates, and candy that ill-informed visitors have brought, unaware that these children have already stopped succumbing to childhood treats. So all the waiting, the fear, the suffering, and the boredom mean these gifts are destined for the parents. Paradoxically, it is outside meal times that the dining room is busier. People pop in again and again throughout the day. This is because there's a small fridge near the window used for storing the bottles of mouthwash—each marked with a child's name—used for preventing ulcers. Although they don't actually eat here, then, the children do come to the dining room for something that gives them hope that they may someday be able to.

At the end of the corridor near the entrance is the playroom. It's a huge space that boasts shelves of books and games, a playhouse, dolls, a tea set, a TV with video games, and a computer. It leads out onto two attractive terraces where the children can play in summer. It's a cheerful, welcoming sort of place. Which is just as well. When they're not feeling too terrible, the children spend hours in here. It's here that they introduce their parents to all sorts of madcap activities: roasting a plastic chicken, looking after a baby doll with cancer, fishing for magnetic fish, piling up wooden rectangles, rolling marbles over a board with holes in it, hiding an aircraft carrier in a corner, riding a scooter over banana skins, and so on. And repeating everything, never-endingly. The parents join in willingly, happy to see their children enjoying themselves. So they get on with it, make mistakes, correct them, and improve. They have fun too sometimes. Most of the time, though, they seem a little absent. Sitting sideways on child-size chairs, with their knees up to their chins, they let their attention and their minds wander until their child calls them to order again. Once a week the activities coordinator suggests a cooking session. Mainly cake making. The children love it. And the parents do too: They don't need to stay. They find themselves with an hour's leave. Back in the playroom, everyone puts on an apron, washes his or her hands, takes a bowl and some flour, yogurt, and sugar. It's a bit like at home, except that here they use liquidized egg that's been pasteurized, just like the milk that comes in cartons. They need to watch out for germs in this apartment.

Entertainment isn't limited to the playroom. It also spills into the corridor, where bikes and trikes are freely available. Being able to make the most of them obviously presupposes the patient doesn't have a drip. This is one way of identifying those who've recently arrived and those preparing to leave: "Unplugged," they celebrate their deliverance by pedaling at breakneck speed. There's also a piano in the corridor that anyone can play. No one can enter or leave the department without brushing past it. It's full of charm, a little worn, in varnished wood with yellowing keys, like an old thing in a saloon bar. There's something strange about this instrument parked here, in among the sick, halfway down a corridor. And what's stranger still is that, despite its dilapidated appearance and the heat in the department, it's more or less in tune. There's no doubting that this piano is tuned regularly. Someone must look after it. So it's not here simply for decorative purposes. People can play it whenever they like and everyone seems to enjoy hearing it. In fact, no one has thought to wedge its soft pedal on. Perhaps that's because not many people actually use it. Solal is in fact one of the few children to use it on a regular basis. To be frank, it's the first thing he does every time he comes back to this apartment. He races over to the velvet-covered stool, puts his hands on the keyboard, and unfailingly tinkles out the first ten bars of the same Tchaikovsky piece. Like a sign of recognition—or of belonging. A nurse or a cleaner can often be heard calling from the far end of the corridor, "I think Solal's back." This makes his parents smile. Then a small group gathers, staff, patients, their families. The caregivers stay on their feet; the parents and children sit on the steps that lead out to the terrace; drips line up, blocking the corridor. They all listen in silence, smiling, moved. It's a great escape.

Very close to the piano, between the bike park and the large picture windows, is one last game. The game. The one that brings together young and old, patients and visitors; the one that causes laughter and bedlam, that takes everyone back to their childhood and makes them forget cancer: table soccer. It's an old design, the sort you still sometimes see in a café. In light-colored wood with red stripes on the sides and blue and red discs to keep the score. Luckily there's an electric socket nearby. Once their pumps are plugged in, the brakes applied to the wheels on their drips, and the tubes secured over their shoulders, the children are completely free to grapple with the handles of those horizontal bars. Suddenly, they're projected inside the stadium, toned as athletes, healthy and sporty, playing alongside their strikers, sweepers, center backs, and goalkeepers. Eleven times more energetic than any healthy person, and eleven times more robust. Untouchable eleven times over. Invincible. After a few months, Solal has become a table soccer grand master. Half-halts, dribbling, knocking back, tackling, spinning—no technique is beyond him. He systematically beats his mother, who, tired of the game or only too glad to make her son happy, adds to her natural incompetence. Solal celebrates every goal. His whoops can be heard on the far side of the department. Oh yes, he's back. There can be a lot of happiness in this apartment.

Farther along the corridor two small terraces allow residents access to the outside. They've recently been reconceived by an architect, the father of a hospitalized child. Each of them is entirely clad in wood and comprises a uniform block constituting a bench with a backrest on either side of a low table. The children don't come out here much—it's not easy climbing up the few steps with a drip. The parents, on the other hand, use them occasionally. They're not allowed to smoke here, for fear the smell will infiltrate the apartment, but these terraces do offer some comfort: escaping the oppressively torrid heat inside, avoiding eye contact with other people, and contemplating the world of the living. Because from up here they have the city at their feet. They can watch normal people living normal lives, rushing to work, missing the bus, carrying bags of shopping, taking children to school and scolding them when they're naughty. Lise likes to choose a passerby at random and follow him or her as far as she can see. She imagines being these other people, takes their every footstep, invents lives for them into which she herself can be subsumed. It isn't to do with making her own life better; in fact, she rarely chooses a mother with healthy-looking children. What she's looking for is difference, not reparation. So she becomes by turns a lovestruck teenage girl, a hurrying businessman, an unsteady old lady, or a rowdy schoolboy. When she's finished bringing to life these flesh-and-blood ghosts, she looks at the world around them. Her gaze cuts across the rue Gay-Lussac, along the rue des Ursulines, picks out the bell tower of Saint-Jacques-du-Haut-Pas Church, takes the rue de l'Abbé-de-l'Épée, and passes the Institute for the Deaf before losing itself in the Luxembourg Gardens that she can only just make out in the distance. Then, cutting diagonally northward, she pictures the boulevard Saint-Michel dropping down to the Seine and the Île de la Cité. The twin towers of Notre-Dame encourage her to look up. She flits over the right bank, and Paris shrinks as if she were a bird on the *wing. Soon, Lise can see the whole city: it isn't a simple entity in white stone and zinc; there's also concrete, metal, brick, tiling, and glass in this agglomeration. The weather is less important to Lise than the fact that time is passing. Perhaps she savors the golden glow of sunlight reflecting off buildings and roofs around her, but bad weather brings its share of light and shade too. It doesn't make any difference: it's just good to breathe the outside air. In this apartment, though, even the terraces fence you in. This is because tall glazed panels have been erected on what should be the open side. They must be well over six feet high, which means the only view is through them. There could have been a guardrail at chest height in wood or cement, hidden with shrubs and flowers. But no. The decision was made to have this insurmountable and coldly transparent wall. Lise can't help thinking about why these glass panels are here; they form far too high a parapet not to be suspect . . . there's a strong chance they're not here simply to prevent accidents. She once found a red balloon abandoned on one of the terraces, and without thinking threw it over the glass wall. She watched it fly away, whisked upward for a moment, and then floating down as if in slow motion and coming to rest softly in the Institute's courtyard, six floors below. There was something rather sad about it lying on the wet asphalt, caught between two green trash cans. Lise stayed there a long time, not moving, with her nose against the glass, reliving that long slow descent, waiting for a breath of wind to free the balloon and bring it to life again. But nothing happened. Tired of waiting, she eventually went back into the apartment, leaving two barely intersecting circles of conden-sation on the glass, like an ephemeral eternity sign.*

The apartment's inhabitants form a strange community. In some ways they are more than roommates, almost family. They didn't choose each other but share an indissoluble sort of existential kinship. A blood tie. In the real sense of the words. Their common ancestor is an aggressive, unstable fellow and they are secret carriers of his unhealthy legacy. He's the psy-chopathic uncle, the Nazi grandfather, the pedophile father. He spawns the unutterable. They meanwhile eat together, sleep together, celebrate Christmas and birthdays, exchange small talk, play, and occasionally laugh, but they avoid talking about this taboo. Tragedy grows in silence. And they all find themselves doubly constrained: they must keep from the others the one thing that should unite them. If they men-tion it they will open up an irreparable breach. No one knows where that might lead. The abyss threatens them all. But hid-ing this evil does nothing to weaken it; in fact, it emerges all the stronger. It wants to be voiced and tries to break down the barriers. And this means that communication between the inhabitants—being subject to the paradoxical injunctions of what can be voiced and what cannot—often revolves around sickness. With the passing days, then, they all harbor iden-tical suffering within them but remain total strangers to each other. In this apartment there's a unique blend of the strange and the familiar.

A CITY

The Institute is a city: it concentrates a dense population in a limited space and provides and facilitates a variety of activities for these citizens. Limited resources mean that everything here is on a miniature scale.

A room of about two hundred square feet therefore serves as a school. As in small rural schools, there's only one class. Two teachers, substitute staff from the national education scheme, welcome students of all abilities and adapt exercises to suit each age group. Primary school children mingle with high-schoolers, and preschoolers with the primary school kids. The school is open every weekday, follows the official curriculum, and respects the calendar of vacations. As such, it is like any other educational establishment in Paris. But in this city, school isn't compulsory, and there are generally few children here. Two or three at the most. Not that it's unpleasant. Quite the opposite, in fact; it's one of the places that connects the children most closely to their previous lives. Which means a lot of them would very much like to attend. Sadly, only too often they're not well enough to do so. It turns out that education, like good health and eating, is one of those privileges we truly value only when deprived of it.

The classroom sometimes also serves as a gymnasium. A sports instructor comes once a week to supervise the children. The chairs are pushed aside, the computers protected, and the only Formica table moved to the middle of the room. It's Ping-Pong time. Traditional bats and balls are used while a piece of string stretched between two yogurt pots acts as a net. The table must be only about five feet long by three feet wide, but that doesn't matter. Its modest dimensions match the physical limitations of the players. In any event, the children wouldn't be able to expend enough energy for normal forms of exercise. Other times there's badminton. Here again, the appropriate type of racket is used but, given the lack of space, the shuttlecock is replaced by a balloon. The children enjoy it, a little. Truth be told, there's something sad, and tragically laughable, about these ersatz sports. The parents probably welcome the organizers' dedication and inventiveness, but they can't help noticing the cramped space, the balls going missing among schoolbooks, rackets getting stuck in pipework, and—as ever—the throwing up that interrupts play. It all seems diminished. Even the children's enjoyment. Parents succumb to a feeling of atrophy and a fear of seeing even this truncated.

Arts and entertainment seem better adapted to the constraints of illness and its treatments. The city has a library that is open to all, consisting of shelves of comics, and there's a media library that boils down to a laptop and a few DVDs. Every now and then a movie theater is set up in the kitchen in the outpatient department on the far side of the main corridor.

*Charlie Chaplin films, Disney films, and a whole selection
of cartoons are screened. Once a week this same kitchen is
transformed into a painting studio. The children give free rein
to their dreams of escape, making this one of the rare occasions when they succeed in forgetting. Lastly, every Tuesday
afternoon, a traveling circus comes to town. It amounts to two
clowns, a man and a woman, with fanciful, brightly colored
clothes, makeup, and red noses. They arrive in a blaze of noise
with booming voices, a barrel organ, tambourines, and party
horns. They go from room to room with a plethora of songs,
jokes, pranks, and magic tricks. They pretend to squabble,
gently castigate the parents, and take the nurses to task while
encouraging the children to side with them. The kids can't get
enough. The adults, meanwhile, are sometimes uncomfortable. They've probably lost that childhood facility for suddenly
changing register. This buffoonery needles and unsettles their
inner trauma. Something about the excesses of farce offends
them. Like the rictus grin of a skull. Whatever the circumstances, the clowns never stray from their roles. From the
moment they step into the city, they are pure comedy and it's
impossible to imagine they have other lives. When they change
back into their everyday clothes, they slip away discreetly
through a hidden door. They never stay around after their
performance. Lise comes across them one evening on their way
out. It takes a while for her to recognize them, stripped of their
artifice. She's not sure who is the more embarrassed, herself or
the two of them.*

For obvious reasons of hygiene, furred and feathered animals as well as plants are banned by municipal law. The city does, however, have a semblance of a zoo and of an indoor jungle. An aquarium with a few aquatic plants and tropical fish has pride of place where the corridors intersect, a point by the entrance to the city that constitutes a sort of traffic circle. But neither the fauna nor the flora appear to flourish here. Confined between ill-lit glass walls and drowning in inadequately oxygenated water, the residents of the zoo are gradually thinning out. After a few months, only mineral and plastic decorations—gravel, rocks, artificial sea wrack, and fake treasure chests—seem to have survived.

The community has no commercial outlets within its walls. Water is dispensed for free in public drinking fountains, but anyone wanting other forms of refreshment or to brighten the day with some extra food must leave the city center and venture into outlying neighborhoods. And this means descending to lower floors, because, thanks to a distinctive feature of local town planning, the city is arranged vertically. It is not until four floors below, then, that you would find a café, which in this instance is called a cafeteria. This single-room establishment is as lacking in charm as it is in visitors, but at least there's the opportunity for several people to meet here to enjoy a cup of tea, a hot chocolate, or a soda, and nibble on an amalgam of saturated fats and rapid-release sugars served up by a machine. It is possible, although rare, to meet people from other neighborhoods here, inhabitants of what the city's residents view as sort of suburbs. And they are a very different population. Older, often less appealing and less cheerful. To tell the truth, the city folk—being fairly protectionist and afraid of being contaminated by foreign sadness—aren't keen to mix with these outsiders. Still, whichever the floor, everyone works in the same sector: medical, paramedical, and peri-medical, and there are only a few paying positions. The city and its suburbs have this feature in common: they both have an unusual number of volunteers.

The city authorities provide residents with a park situated on the very periphery of the suburbs at street level. Here citizens can meet inhabitants of the whole conurbation, patients, caregivers, and administrators. But the children don't go there often; it's hard to get down the stairs out to the garden with a chemo drip. And there's not much to do there, anyway. You can't play soccer or racket games or leapfrog. It's mostly populated by adults who are here to smoke. Gardening workshops are sometimes held for the children, and this means putting on gloves because those in aplasia are not allowed to touch the soil. And anyway this presupposes that they are strong enough and feel like going outside. Which is rare in cases of aggressive treatments such as Solal's. And, when it comes down to it, if they're venturing outside, they'd prefer to be going home. In this miniature city, confinement comes as standard. People don't often set foot outside, except to leave. The population is secretly haunted by dreams of an urban exodus. Each individual understands that the whole community is just an illusion in the middle of a very real city whose heart beats to the rhythm of real life.

BABEL

The Institute is a tower in the middle of Paris. It's a citadel, a fortress erected on the topmost floor of a building, on the heights of the hill known as the Montagne Sainte-Geneviève. Within its closed walls, it looks down over the plains like the Hanging Gardens of Babylon. From the summit there are views over the urban expanse spreading at its feet, like the sea at the foot of a cliff. The viewer can picture the curve of the horizon in the distance where the sphere of the earth drops away. But hardly anyone ventures that far, even in their imagination.

This is because up on that promontory, in the sealed world of the pediatric oncology department, different geodetics preside. It is a confined flat shape, like the earthly disc of the Ancients. It has clearly defined limits, four corners and edges. No need to look elsewhere. It is the one and only measure of the universe, sufficient unto itself.

This tower is an entire world. A microcosm develops within it, constituting a scaled-down planet. People here are from all over the place, although predominantly France, Africa, and eastern Europe. The whole world seems to have agreed to meet in this little scrap of space. *Inheritors of a mixed-race people and temporary beneficiaries of a host nation, a heterogeneous people gathers here with no distinctions of class, color, origin, or faith. It's a melting pot of humanity. There are hijabs, bubus, kippahs, and ushankas. Crosses, stars, hands, and lotuses. The food is kosher, halal, vegetarian, and vegan. There's fasting for Yom Kippur, Lent, and Ramadan. At Christmas everyone decorates the tree in the reception area and hopes for presents. When the time comes for Eid the same people share cakes made with honey, pistachio, and orange flower water. For the Sabbath, meatballs and challah bread are handed around. Sometimes the scent of spices, incense, and patchouli in the corridors even drowns out the astringent smell of antiseptics. The Institute reinvents republican universalism and practices it in its own way. It establishes an expanded, open, plural France. It relaxes her insistence on secularity, calls chiefly for equality of treatment and fraternity in the fight, and authorizes multiculturalism and the expression of different faiths. Only the citizens' liberty is open to question, and this is because freedom in this world does not depend on others. Here cancer is supreme sovereign.*

The inhabitants of the tower mostly get along well. They could even be said to understand each other. Although they don't all have the same mother tongue. Some have no mastery of French. The diagnoses, treatments, recommendations, and conversations must adapt to this diversity. The place is, by its very nature, multilingual. On December 31, a large sheet *of white paper is circulated and each parent writes "Happy New Year" in different-colored felt pens and in the language of his or her choice. There's Arabic, Russian, Fula, Creole, Serb, Kabyle, Romanian, Vietnamese, and Portuguese. The variety of wordings, alphabets, and colors creates an exuberant patchwork that helps all concerned forget that this year doesn't look set to be particularly happy. Despite the language barriers and the confined living space, there are few disagreements and misunderstandings. Tolerance prevails. This is because, over and above the differences in origin, everyone does share a common language. It is a living, growing cross-border language, a complex idiom made up of linguistic, vocal, graphic, and gestural signs. It has its realia, metaphors, and expressions, its rituals and dialects. It has simple grammar, extremely precise technical vocabulary, and endless lexical expanses dealing with sensations and feelings. It frequently uses imagery, but rarely conjugation: its users mostly confine themselves to the present, avoiding the past and the future. Although incidents of the conditional have been reported, the indicative is the predominant mode. It belongs to a family of ancestral languages: they have been used in different forms for millennia to express suffering. There are no manuals for them. This language cannot be taught or studied; its users are only ever self-taught. Besides, it is rarely expressed in oral or written form, because users appear to prefer limiting themselves to gestural signs. Its use is therefore recognized in an exchange of eye contact, a hand on a shoulder, a hug, a smile, or a silence. Although freshly coined and mostly tacit, it still allows for members of the group to identify with each other and communicate. As if affording a kind of union to all these disparate individuals who are—in spite of themselves—involved in a shared promethean enterprise. As if the people of Babel have pooled their strength to reach the top of the tower at last. But however civilized the place may be, no one can forget that it stands on a dangerous fault line.*

I IS ANOTHER

L ise doesn't talk about her situation. Ever. She never says, "It's horrible," "It's not fair," "It's unbearable." Or even, "I'm so unlucky," "I'm frightened," or simply "It hurts." She discusses neither what has happened, nor what will happen, what might happen, what should have happened, or what could have happened. In front of other people, she avoids the ifs, in every tense and mood. All that counts is the present. Only current facts are entitled to be expressed: "Solal's eating," "Solal's sleeping," "Solal's throwing up," "Solal's playing," "Solal's laughing," "Solal's crying," "Solal's in pain." That's the state of affairs and that's it. Still, there must be questions, doubts, and hypotheses somewhere, but in such a forbidden version of reality that they have no access to language. They remain implicit, incommunicable. Her "I" is kept firmly shut.

Lise doesn't think about her situation. Ever. She doesn't think, "It's horrible," "It's not fair," "It's unbearable." Or even, "I'm so unlucky," "I'm frightened," or simply "It hurts." She doesn't wonder what's happened, or what will happen, what might happen, what should have happened, or what could have *happened. Even with herself, she avoids the ifs, in every tense and mood. All that counts is the present. Only current facts are entitled to be considered. Solal's eating, Solal's sleeping, Solal's throwing up, Solal's playing, Solal's laughing, Solal's crying, or Solal's in pain. That's the state of affairs and that's it. Still, there must be questions, doubts, and hypotheses somewhere, but in such a deeply buried version of reality that it has no access to thought. It remains latent, larval. Her "I" is kept firmly covered.*

Lise doesn't feel her situation. Most of the time she feels nothing at all. Not the horror, not the unfairness, the suffering, or the rebellion. She doesn't experience; she simply does. She's just a series of actions, a collection of functions. Tending, washing, feeding, consoling, entertaining. Her only form is verbal. She no longer has a name. As if being a mother to the extreme has ended up removing her from her own existence. This is what she has become: a force that does what needs to be done. Leaning forward, eyes determined, words and gestures carefully measured, she gives herself entirely to her child. She seems to plow forward like this ahead of herself, leaving her true self behind. She never turns around to see how she's doing. Whether she's managing to keep up. Or is just still there. She never thinks to and never has an opportunity to. Her identity is being lost along the way as she strays in the space between a me and a someone else.

Sometimes, although rarely, Lise talks to the other mothers about cancer. About the cancer their children have, not her

*child's. In the early days she deliberately avoided all contact
with them. She knew that empathy comes naturally to her and
didn't want to risk deflecting it from its target. She needed to
focus wholeheartedly on her son. There was no room for other
people's children. Then time passed, the Institute became more
familiar, the treatments more effective, the side effects better handled, and Solal more autonomous; and Lise found she
was thinking about the world around her again. And listening
to it. She met some people, established connections that were
both distant and peculiarly close. At first she would automatically steer conversations to everyday topics: the weather, how
the department was run, the food, whether the rooms were
clean. Just describing the facts, again. She was wary. And
quite rightly, because gradually snatches of personal experience insinuated themselves into the other women's words. Once
there was a feeling of trust, their words grew freer, became
more detailed and specific. Now they open their hearts to her.
Some are clearly suffering from a deficiency, a need to tell
their story like this, for want of anyone to talk to. For want of
listeners, mostly. The outside world doesn't understand them,
they've lost their friends, they're afraid of psychologists, their
husbands have fled, figuratively and, sadly, sometimes also
literally. The Institute is mostly a women's story. And so it is
that a couple of mothers end up describing their extended torture to Lise, their own private stations of the cross that they've
endured since the first signs of their child's sickness. Their accounts are long-winded, intense, and blunt while also detailed*

and well informed. Under control. Their words ring true; their sentences string together naturally; their voices don't crack. In describing their devastation, these women have invented a descriptive style that is cool and yet still laden with fear, rage, and despair. The absence of pathos in these bleakest of circumstances is chilling. Like a stifled death rattle coming from a calm, sterilized room. As she listens to them, Lise thinks no one should have to suffer this much; no human being is designed to withstand this. Their minds won't hold out. Madness lies in wait. And when their minds come undone, it's their bodies that will fail: the wombs that carried and bore these children will explode, laying bare insides devoted only to the agonies of delivery, insides that cannot tolerate the premature decline of creatures that, by their very essence, should survive them. Lise feels indignation, pity, and sympathy for these women. She suffers on their behalf. She even sometimes weeps at the thought of their iniquitous fate.

Once, just once, Lise is struck by the thought of herself. Thunderstruck by it. Isn't she, in fact, exactly like these women whom she pities with all her heart? She is here with them. And for the same reason. Day after day she too experiences all the things in their lives that she finds horrifying. She too has had the news, the waiting, the failures, the mistakes, the shocks, the scandals, the improvements, and the relapses. She too is going through the stations of the cross. She too is confronted with the intolerable. She's one of them. She's like them. It's so crudely, so stupidly obvious that Lise doesn't understand how she can have turned her back on it for such a long time. The idea is both so self-evident and so utterly ignored that it's almost absurd. Lise needs to dwell on this awhile, to stop herself smiling about it. And only then does the savage, naked truth hit her. She feels. She doesn't directly experience the torments of her true self. Her "I" is still another woman. There needs to be an intermediary. So yes, she feels but by proxy, by transitivity. Or through syllogism: these women are suffering; she is like them; she must therefore be suffering. Either way, she does now feel pain at last. Pain for the woman she is, who must go through such an ordeal. Pain for the woman who needs to fight every waking moment to save her mind from madness and her insides from exploding. Pain for herself, for Lise. The tears that now flow are almost sweet. But Lise can't linger here. Having barely glimpsed herself, she must move on already. Yes, she absolutely must keep going. There is so much to do and Solal needs her.

PHOTOGRAPHS

I could write. Keep a sort of journal, describe what's happening day-to-day, explore my feelings. Keep a record of passing time. I could do that but I don't want to or have time to. It doesn't feel appropriate for the Institute. Too slow and painstaking. And too reflective. Because in order to write about the present I would, paradoxically, need to extricate myself from it, and that sort of distance proves impossible. Materially at first: I have so much to do for you that I wouldn't find the time to write. And if and when I can free myself for a few hours, benefiting from a rare morning when you're asleep or an afternoon when you don't feel nauseous, I very much doubt I'd have the inner reserves for it. Writing assumes a degree of vacancy, not only in our actions but also in the mind. I don't have the type of leisurely freedom here that makes a diarist. Even the waiting, even the boredom, even the emptiness are filled with you. And, to be honest, I'm not sure I'd have much to gain from it. It could even prove dangerous. I mean, who knows what might happen if I started thinking about my experience? I think my strength relies on too much obliviousness to take a risk like that.

And yet I'm afraid of forgetting. Not the first days, of course, that have been inscribed into my flesh by the whirlwind chronology of catastrophe, but the ensuing weeks and months, when the extraordinary settles so naturally into routine that it eventually dissolves into it. Yes, I'm afraid, afraid I'll forget the names, dates, events, places, people, emotions, and, worse still, sensations. I don't want it all to disappear before we've even had an opportunity to scrutinize it. It would be like a crime without a trial. An abominable hit-and-run. The kind that robs victims of their status and allows for every sort of revisionism. Whatever the outcome, I don't want what has happened not to have existed for any of us. There's a vital insistence to this fear; a hope, if not necessarily for a happy outcome, at least for a much-needed reconstruction. The villain, the stealthy infanticide, has struck. Is still striking. Will perhaps win. But its misdeeds won't go unpunished. It will have to answer for each of its acts. I'll draw up a list, confront the villain with the truth, investigate the crime myself, and file the case for you, for your brother and sister, for your father, for myself and all the others. This is how it has to be. So many things could stop me achieving this, the usual after-effects of trauma: inertia, inhibition, collapse, avoidance, and amnesia. I'm particularly wary of a kind of emotional contagion in which we over-adapt to horror to the point of denying its existence and even liking the very thing that hurts us. Stockholm syndrome. I'm frightened all this will stop us living fully again one day, or is pushing the deadline for that life so far into the future that it will be too late. The adults will be too old and the children too adult. I'm worried about this statute of limitations.

The decision is made. I'm opening the file. Right now. And because I can't work out how to write, I'll settle for gathering evidence. I have the perfect tool for this: the camera on my iPhone. With that I can capture visual evidence in real time, compile it, and save it for later analysis. Images rather than words, that's the solution. Images are good; they're direct, instant, and apparently neutral. They can claim to be objective. Of course, there's always a point of view, a particular angle, but this can be kept discreet, giving the observer an impression of mimicry. This isn't commentary, merely observation. And it avoids the rift created by language, the unbridgeable gap between words and things. Because I fully understand that it's there, through this breach that meaning escapes, that feelings, uncertainties, and ambiguities creep in. All the things that make up a text in its fragility and instability. All the things I don't have it in me to confront right now. And so I choose images. I won't be a diarist; I'll be a photojournalist. I'll collect photos, will superimpose them onto one another, erecting a tower to fight the tendency to forget. They can be the modest recollections of my soul, palimpsests of memory resisting any erosion. My own miniature pyramid.

Some days, when the conditions are right, I photograph like crazy: the department, objects, the atmosphere. People less so. And definitely not the patients. Too intrusive. I'd feel I was violating their privacy. But their presence is still felt in the images. They implicitly inhabit the department and use the objects, giving them form and meaning. There's a strong sense of how full of life it all is; life, love, conversations, ordeals, pain, struggles, rebellion, and acceptance. There's humanity even in kidney-shaped bowls, in the diaphragms on pumps, in the valves on tubes. So many people are implied by these things: The biologists' work, the technicians' dexterity, the oncologists' decisions, the nurses' care. You can also infer the parents' concern, the commitment of all the staff, the motivation of a team. Lastly, you can deduce a sense of childhood, the joy, the games, the suffering, the pain, the exhaustion, and the calls for help.

Sometimes I film too, and record sounds. The steady A-note of alarms, sixty strident beats per minute, the muted creaking sound of injected fluids, like the boards of an old boat reverberating to the regular smack of water. A lot of people probably think it strange of me to be capturing the unspeakable, apparently coldly and unthinkingly, when it should be enough for me to experience it. They would most likely understand better if I committed it to paper in secret at a desk. The time for writing is bound to come. For now, I'm establishing my audiovisual archives, and stockpiling

my snapshots. It's my way of securing the present in order
to check the inevitable flow of time. And perhaps this compulsive hoarding is also to ward off the terror of losing you.
A delusion, an ironic sort of carpe diem. I genuinely don't
intend to put captions on these photos later; I just hope that
someday they'll help mitigate the gaps in my inadequate
memory.

I don't yet know that I'll never actually see these photos again. Not that I'll lose them, but because I won't feel
up to facing them. I'll be too scared of being confronted
with the image of you in your weakened state. Because I
do sometimes take pictures of you. The way people simply
do photograph their children. As if you weren't ill. To hold
on to a happy moment, a visit from a friend, your favorite
nurse, little Emma who became your "Curie sister," a performance you improvised, or a game you invented. Or just
because I think you look beautiful with your close-cropped
hair. One day, in three years' time, thanks to a text conversation, I'll chance across a few of these snapshots that
I sent to a friend. And they'll cause terror. I'll see nothing but the abomination of it: the morphine in the nurse's
hand, the needle in Emma's shoulder, the awkwardness in
your friend's smile. Your face will reveal the distortions due
to cortisone, your scalp, the loss of hair, and your eyes, a
terrible distress. I'll think you look ugly, deformed, unbearable to behold. It will all come crashing back: first the
smells, then the sounds, tastes, sensations. My stomach will

be gripped with panic. My legs will falter. My head will spin. And then I'll think of the hundred or so other secretly stored images. I'll imagine them suddenly coming back to life, using any opportunity to escape from their archives, like a strong wind that's been kept at bay but barges inside the moment a door is opened. I'll imagine them organizing themselves into a wild tornado, swirling in a funnel around me, tearing me off the floor of the apartment and flinging me, broken and inert, in some abandoned place. No, for sure, I'll never see these pictures. I won't open any doors to them. They'll stay sensibly shut away in their digital file. Enclosed, buried, like a tomb that no one ever visits and yet they think of it often.

It's a photo among plenty of others. Backlit. It shows a wooden table-soccer table in front of two huge windows. The table's legs lean slightly so that they fit perfectly in the bottom corners of the photo and seem destined to meet at some vanishing point in the upper half. There's a child sitting under the table, cross-legged, straight-backed, his hands on his knees. He is bald. He's facing the windows with his back to the photographer. He's wearing roomy pajamas, and a tube emerges from them and leads off to some unidentified place out of shot. The whole setup has its own strange aesthetic. Is it the contrast between the light-filled background and the underexposed foreground that lends a black-and-white quality to the colors, dissolving living and inanimate things in half-darkness? Is it the rigorous construction of the image that endorses the child's presence so symmetrically, almost concentrically? Impossible to say. In any event, it produces mixed emotions. At first glance, it captivates with a sort of serenity. Protected by the wooden structure, silent and motionless in the lotus position, with his shaven head and delicate body, the child looks like a meditating bonze. A Buddha in his stupa. It's not hard to imagine the great sage's contemplative smile on the child's unseen face. And yet the picture demands a second reading. Its very peacefulness gives rise to a sense of melancholy. Something cracks. Like a cruel, ill-defined fault line carved into that calm, ordered world. Perhaps it's just nostalgia. The empty playroom implies the end of childhood. Perhaps it's something else, something that must remain unspoken. Whatever the case, Lise feels that of all the photos taken at the Institute, this one definitely comes closest to the reality of it.

VISITS

O ther than their parents and brothers and sisters, the young patients have few visitors. From the start the oncologists recommend choosing potential visitors carefully and sparingly. Contrary to expectations, hygiene isn't the only reason for this. Granted, chemotherapy produces substantial drops in immune defenses, and, with more aggressive treatments like Solal's, there can be repeated periods of total aplasia. But the risk of contamination is there even with no external contact. True danger comes from inside. Every child actually has a cargo of germs in his or her body, keen to multiply if and when the shield of white cells weakens. So when the polynuclear neutrophil count drops toward zero, the patient can self-contaminate. Which means that a visit from a friend with the flu, a fever, or any other contagious complaint would only accelerate an inevitable process. In aplasia, patients systematically end up developing infections and then need emergency antibiotics to avoid septicemia. Cancer's way of confirming that in adversity we are all our own worst enemy. When the medical team encourage limiting visitors, then, it's more to do with the inherent demands of the treatment and the

patients' subsequent weakness. Often bedridden, tired, nau-
seous, and subjected to repeated interventions by nurses, these
children barely have a moment's respite. Although it's import-
ant that they maintain contact with their old lives, there are no
guarantees that they'll be able to cope with this contact while
they're at the Institute. Which is why the question of visitors
isn't merely a physiological consideration. During visits chil-
dren can be overwhelmed by negative emotions: first, shame
for their bodies that no longer belong to them—their hairless
heads, the uncontrolled vomiting, the loss of bladder control
and sometimes loss of bowel control; frustration too that they
can't make the most of a visit; and, last, a longing for this
other world from which they feel excluded, and a feeling of
rebellion precisely because they are excluded.

Visitors' personalities must also be taken into account.
How close they are to the child, how well they will handle the
situation, whether they can cope with another person's suf-
fering. Because friends visiting the Institute are also exposed
to a form of contamination. No one enters a pediatric oncol-
ogy department without taking risks, particularly if they're
ten years old. There are plenty of endemic factors: seeing a
friend's physical decline, being confronted with other sick chil-
dren who may be maimed or deformed, realizing that lives
are at stake, even the hospital surroundings, the sounds and
smells, the inertia. Young visitors are also threatened with a
loss of innocence. So it's all a question of choice and timing.
Well chosen and scheduled at the right time, a visitor can have

positive effects: providing a distraction, laughter and happiness, maintaining a sense—if not of normality—at least of continuity, reinforcing the fighting spirit, giving new hope. But the opposite can also be true, condemning all concerned to acute disappointment and sorely testing the friendship. As a result, only one rule applies: the patient chooses who he or she would like to see, and when. The parents make the arrangements. Most of the time Solal prefers to wage his battle out of sight of the outside world. Illness has its own propriety. Still, in the first and last days of each round of chemotherapy when the side effects are less apparent, he sometimes agrees to see the few willing visitors among his friends, cousins, aunts, and uncles. Those closest to him, perhaps those who will best withstand it too. But after a few months, one constant becomes apparent; a sort of tacit law that operates independently of the patient's own wishes seems to govern every visit. If you are neither the parent nor the grandparent of a hospitalized child, you come to the Institute only once. With very rare exceptions, no one asks to come back.

ESTELLE

I t all starts with a good intention. The road to hell is paved
with them, as everyone knows. The idea is to cheer up
Solal's second day in the hospital by allowing him to spend
a few hours with Nathan, who's been his best friend at school
for more than seven years. It's not only a commendable idea, but
also feasible, because the treatment doesn't yet have any visible
side effects. Solal's strength, immune defenses, appetite, diges-
tion, hair, and enthusiasm are all still intact. So Lise has happily welcomed this suggestion from her friend Estelle, Nathan's
mother. Any form of distraction is good for the taking, so long
as it's practicable. And from that point of view it's a success:
the boys are playing table soccer in the corridor, having a great
time. In Solal's room, it's a different story. The two women are
engaged in a precarious conversation. Estelle has sat herself on
the edge of Solal's bed and for a good ten minutes she's been
intent on proving to Lise how run-of-the-mill her situation is.
Or perhaps she wants to prove it to herself. She's trying to reassure someone, anyway. Estelle wants Lise to tell her she's not
afraid, and doggedly encourages her to make this pronounce-
ment with a battery of rhetorical questions and denials: "You're

EXODUS

not worried, though, are you? What do you think's going to happen? Everything seems to be going fine." Lise doesn't know what to say. Of course she's worried, but that's not the problem, and there's no point wrangling over it. Unlike Estelle, she feels no need to comfort herself by minimizing the battle. She's already assessed its importance, its every phase and risk, what the chances are and what's at stake. She's been told the treatment will be tough. It will be. She's been told it will be long. It will be. She's been told that victory is possible but not guaranteed. Duly noted. Lise has bowed to the inevitable. She's looked the enemy in the face, chosen her camp, and rolled up her sleeves. All she's interested in now are the facts. She utters a hesitant "Well, yes I am, but we're going to win," intended single-handedly to limit outpourings of subjectivity. But Estelle doesn't see it like that. "Look," she says, "your boy's full of life, he's playing, he's absolutely fine." Lise explains reluctantly that it won't go on like this, the chemo will have side effects and it's better to be forewarned. "Oh, but that's nothing," Estelle replies. "He can just rest when he's tired and then he'll be cured. It's no big deal. There's nothing to worry about." Now this really is getting difficult. It needs to stop. "Listen," Lise retorts, "he'll get the best possible treatment here, sure. There are risks, it'll take a long time, and sometimes it'll be hard, but we have plenty of grounds for hope. We're doing what needs to be done and that's all there is to it." This still doesn't seem to be enough: "You know my son could die too. When he walks out of here he could be run over by a car. The risks are the same for everyone.

201

*It's not all about you." Lise is lost for words. She contemplates
various possibilities: a statistical demonstration, a psychological analysis, philosophical reflections, or a direct attack. But
she doesn't have the energy for any of these, so she goes for the
easiest option and chooses escape: "I'm going to get a glass of
water. Would you like one?"*

Sitting on the steps to the terrace with my cup in my hand,
I watch the boys playing table soccer. It's a happy interlude;
they're having a good time. Solal doesn't even seem to be
hampered by the pole, the tube, the drip pump, and the electric cable. He whoops with each goal scored. To be frank, he's
over the moon. Estelle comes to sit next to me. She must be
tired of waiting for her glass of water. She leans toward me,
takes my hand, and in a quiet voice laden with emotion, says:
"Can I ask you a favor?" "Yes, of course," I reply, privately
wondering if she wants me to help her son cross the road.
Not far wrong, in fact. "Could you look after Nathan for an
hour or two?" I accept. Particularly graciously, in fact, because I was planning to make the most of this absence of side
effects to go for a half-hour run in the Luxembourg Gardens.
There won't be many more opportunities like this. Solal is
fine, the medical team are keeping an eye on him, they're big
boys, they can play happily while they wait for their mothers
to come back. My reply, although positive, doesn't appear to

suit Estelle. She was expecting something else. The fact is, she was expecting me to probe her, which, given her tone of voice, struck me as a very bad idea. Unabashed, Estelle goes ahead and answers the unformulated question. "It's, well, I need to visit someone on the fifth floor, someone whose wife..." Her voice cracks. Conspicuously. I don't say anything. Estelle can keep waiting. Tiring of the wait, she continues: "...whose wife is in this hospital and she's, she's..." Another sob. Another silence. I keep my counsel. I can see clearly where this is going, and I don't want to know any more. I'm definitely not a helpful person to talk to. "Darn it, I'll have to do this all by myself," Estelle must be thinking. "...she's dying of cancer." Tears, shaking, voice falling apart. This may seem strange but I secretly want to laugh. Now it's my turn to take her hand. "It must be someone you're very close to for you to be so upset." Having bad things happen to us doesn't make us nice people. It makes me if not sarcastic, at least ironic. I know her family is fine: her only son is right here in front of my eyes, she has no brothers and sisters, her parents are so healthy they exhaust her, her husband left her, and she doesn't go out much. Still, it has to be said that I've finally consented to ask a sort of question. Estelle makes the most of this and replies tearfully, as if this were ultimate proof of the agonizing fate being visited on her: "He's a customer at the pharmacy where I work." "Yes, poor you, that must be very hard. I'm going to get my sneakers." Escape is my best ally once again.

———

*It's nice out in the Luxembourg Gardens with glorious sun-
shine warming the chill December air, and Lise is not the only
person running. She congratulates herself for this very pleas-
ant escape. Truth be told, she's surprised and amused to find
some comfort here, because of all the sports she's ever tried,
jogging is perhaps her least favorite. She doesn't feel strong
enough mentally for it. She likes running only if she's pursuing
something. She needs something to run for: a tennis ball, a
soccer ball, a shuttlecock. It sets up an exchange and that's
what makes the game. Having no tangible goal and being
fundamentally solitary, running requires too much discipline,
which she feels comes close to masochism. She's tried her hand
at it, though, over very modest distances, six miles maximum.
But she soon gets bored. Like a lot of people, she started running with earphones so music could serve as entertainment. It
worked for a while, but the disconnect between what she was
hearing and her other senses soon bothered her. She then tried
pacing her stride to match the exact rhythm of whatever she
was listening to. Every three and a half minutes or thereabouts
a different song would come along and change the parameters
of her running: the frequency of her strides, her arm movements, and her breathing. The results were more entertaining
for other people than for herself. Besides the psychomotor limitations of the exercise, the music itself ended up annoying her.
She claimed it not only stopped her appreciating the natural*

world around her but also forced her to listen to her own paces. Concentrating on every breath and every footfall, and ensuring they were in time with each other, became the sole objectives of her jogging. Feeling an internal rhythm and melting into it, finding where she belonged in this fickle reality. Once this had happened there was no question of being distracted.

Today, of course, the problem has presented itself slightly differently. It was certainly more appropriate than ever to escape her fears and concerns with a concrete form of activity, and this was what had persuaded Lise to bring her sneakers to the Institute this morning. But her run in the public gardens ended up serving an unexpected purpose: escaping Estelle. As she has a quick wash in the bathroom attached to Solal's room and listens to him and Nathan playing cards on his bed, Lise decides that jogging does actually have its upsides.

When she starts drying herself with paper towels, Lise hears adult voices in the bedroom. The first, a woman's voice, she thinks she can identify as Cécile, one of Solal's nurses. The second, a man's, is unfamiliar. Driven by intuition, Lise rushes through her drying process and comes out to join the boys. Sure enough, Cécile is there, hanging a chemotherapy pouch on top of the pole, while the boys keep playing their card game without batting an eyelid. At the foot of the bed is a frail old man with a mustache talking to the nurse. And next to him is Estelle. The nurse looks embarrassed but Lise doesn't have time to wonder why, because the man turns to talk to her: "Hi there. Did you realize we live in the same building? Isn't that funny." Lise doesn't understand. She doesn't know who this man is nor what he's doing in her son's bedroom. She's just vaguely uncomfortable, like when something simply feels wrong. The mustache, maybe. Seeing her bafflement, the visitor tries again: "We live in the same building, you're on staircase A, I think, and I'm on staircase F. Estelle told me." Lise still doesn't understand. The man persists, probably thinking her rather obtuse. "Well, it's a funny coincidence, we live in the same place and you're here with your son and me with my wife on the fifth floor. She also has cancer and she's..." This time Lise gets it. Well, the man did give her a clue. He formulated his words in exactly the same way as Estelle. As if dying constituted an activity that always needed to be expressed in the present progressive. She personally doesn't find this particularly "funny." And she certainly has no intention of letting him finish this sentence in front of Solal. She cuts right across him: "Excuse me, but I'd prefer to go somewhere else to discuss this. It's nothing to do with the children." Truth be told, it's nothing to do with her either.

In the corridor Lise explains quietly that they've been advised to limit the number of visitors and it therefore makes sense to restrict them to people whose presence really means something to the child. She adds that she's very sorry to hear about the man's wife, but she doesn't think it desirable to mention her imminent death in front of her child. The man appears to understand and beats a retreat. Estelle escorts him to the elevators and then returns. She takes big strides, her chest puffed out, comes to stand squarely in front of Lise, and spits viciously, "That was so rude, what you just did. I didn't think you were that kind of person." Lise explains again. Just in case Estelle still doesn't understand the context. Her friend is getting angry. She's very red in the face and throws her arms around convulsively. She looks as though she might take off. Sadly, she doesn't. What she actually does is start yelling. Lise is very embarrassed. Not because she drove away Mr. Mustache, but by her friend's behavior. There are dozens of parents in the department whose children are very sick, in danger, and in some cases may even be doing that same present-progressive thing. But there are never any raised voices here. No one ever complains, sobs, or screams in this corridor. Everyone respects everyone else's pain and makes no great display of their own. It isn't a written law. It's just the way it is. A question of manners. Or survival. So Lise is ashamed; she feels at fault for bringing into the Institute a woman who's disturbing the precious equilibrium of the place. She should have seen this coming. Right now what she needs to do is contain the scene and not succumb to anger herself. She has better things to do. Luckily, her fight against cancer has mobilized all her resources and therefore forbids her sacrificing even the smallest part of them to anything inessential. Luckily again, Olivier appears at this point. Lise hastily summarizes the situation for him and asks him to get rid of this nuisance. Olivier has no energy to spare either so he reacts instantly. He instinctively takes Estelle by the shoulders, physically containing her outburst, while begging her, gently but firmly, to leave *the inpatient department. There in the reception area, in front of the elevators, he then suffers several long minutes of verbal incontinence that, despite his own steady entreaties, he doesn't succeed in stemming. Estelle whines, curses, yells, and shrieks. She keeps on and on saying, "You're not the only ones with problems. I have issues too." Her screams carry to the far end of the department. Olivier stands firm. Lise can't hear what he's saying to Estelle but knows he has it in him not to blow his top. And is reassured by this. She sits down on the yellow sofa in the corridor. Cécile comes to sit next to her and puts a hand tactfully on Lise's arm.*

"What you've just been put through is very tough," she says. "I felt terrible for you. There was nothing you could have done, you know, it happens sometimes. Anyway, you reacted very well. There was no other way to handle it."

Lise savors the dual comforts of Cécile's gesture and her words. Other than this, she doesn't feel anything much at all. Not anger, hate, disgust, regret, or even exhaustion. She is simply grateful to Cécile and Olivier for their support and hopes she can return to normality as soon as possible. But for several hours to come she will have a subtle trembling sensation in her limbs.

Two days later Lise receives a text from Estelle. She apologizes for her behavior. She doesn't even understand it herself. It's frank and direct; it's all Lise needs. She forgives her and immediately forgets about it. Estelle never visited the Curie again.

ACCOMPANIST

There is one man among Lise and Olivier's friends who comes to the Institute regularly. He's Simon, Solal's piano teacher. Right from the first week of treatment he arrives at the hospital every Saturday at the exact time that the child usually has his lesson at home. This arrangement happened almost of its own accord. Lise thought it would be good for Solal, who proved enthusiastic about the idea. When they asked Simon whether he would be happy with it, he immediately accepted. Now everyone behaves as if this is simply a change of address, and over time the benefits of this weekly visit turn out to be considerable. In the first instance this is due to the very act of playing music, which doubly fulfills the task of keeping the child occupied. On the one hand, the piano captures all his attention and focuses it on specific things—reading the score, respecting the rhythm, and accuracy on the keyboard; on the other, it releases his imagination and invites it to escape. By the end of the session this repeated sequence of contractions and relaxations produces a sort of vital flow, rather as the cardiac muscle does. The artistic element remains somewhat limited at the Institute, though, and this is because *medical circumstances always end up gaining the upper hand. Most of the time, Solal isn't strong enough to play or even to stay sitting at the piano for the whole lesson. On his best days the lesson lasts no more than thirty minutes. And even then, while Simon beats out the rhythm, adjusts the position of Solal's hands, or corrects a wrong note, he has to keep a spare kidney bowl on his knees, ready to position it between the child and the keyboard at the slightest sign of retching. The fact is unavoidable and is accepted as such. Vomit breaks are now part of the lesson's routine, as the chocolate break once was. The pedagogic limitations don't really matter much. Every note played and every chord achieved in itself constitutes a sort of victory over the cancer, one that is both minor and essential. It makes the possibility of forgetting into something tangible. Besides the musical content, Simon's presence here is enough to reconstitute hope. By keeping up this Saturday ritual, he lends a familiar pattern to the weeks in the hospital, he simulates ordinary life and introduces a semblance of normality into this oncological exception. And so a simple music lesson enshrines evidence of continuity above the chaos.*

Solal is not the only one to benefit from this visit; his mother draws comfort from it too. This is because Simon is more than a piano teacher; he also accompanies the songs that Lise has been writing, composing, and performing for a number of years. It means they have a special understanding. A piano doesn't simply follow the voice; it supports it, carries it, gives it solid reference points along its way like stepping stones across a river. Every note can then find where to alight with confidence. This technical constancy guarantees freedom in the interpretation. On the rhythmic and harmonic base provided by the instrument, Lise picks out her path and grants herself variations. She invents, allowing nuances, high notes, and the tempo to fluctuate. The tune wavers, steps out of line, trips, and bounces back. These small discrepancies aren't merely ornamental, they introduce a suspense that gives the piece its true identity. Because agreeing to take a step to the side means risking losing her footing. It's never safe. It takes so little— one eighth note too many, one ill-timed semitone, one forgotten quarter rest—and everything can end up in the water. From an artistic point of view, this danger is an asset: the listener quivers with fearful anticipation of a fall, but these falls are rarely truly damaging. Professional accompanists can save the day; they have tricks up their sleeves. The hiatus of uncertainty when instrument and singer appear to diverge irretrievably only increases the pleasure when they're reunited, and these reconquered harmonies produce pleasurable emotions. Even so, Simon isn't happy simply supporting the melody on the piano; he too makes digressions. He adapts, adds color, ornaments with counterpoints, motifs and leitmotifs, other voices, and even other instruments. He also alters the silences, often inhabiting them discreetly with the softest arpeggio or with pearlescent notes whispered into this musical darkness. Or he prepares for them with such a furtive diminuendo that it eventually melts into absence. But he also sometimes lengthens

them. Aided and abetted like this, every song is a wonderful
opportunity to escape, and it's a narrow escape. It's a break-
away that, wherever it may wander, is bound to end happily.

Needless to say, there are no opportunities for such escapes
at the Institute. The endless comings and goings of nurses and
visitors, the hiss and bleep of machines, the presence of sick
children, the very ugliness of their illness, and most of all the
fear skulking in the shadows—everything here constrains and
inhibits creativity. Lise, who was so prolific the year before,
has actually stopped composing since she was told that Solal
has cancer. She no longer has the time or the inclination for
it. It's not something she thought about. It's just what happened. Her inspiration dried up in the same way that it arrived, spontaneously, instinctively. Before, it would well up of
its own accord. For no apparent reason, Lise would feel something bubbling to the surface, a brief phrase or a few words
accompanied by succinct notes. Then she sat at the piano and,
through the successions of chords, she allowed these tributary
motifs to converge into other, more substantial flows. The melody then expanded, picking out the contours of a story as it
found its course. That's all over for now. No more notes and
no more words. None of it. Lise simply has nothing left to say.
But having Simon here still makes her want to sing. Unable
to compose anything new together, the two friends choose to
revive existing material. In the barren desert to which cancer
confines them, covers of famous songs stand in for creativity.
They alight on familiar material and add their own unusual

nuances of stitch and color. They improvise. With its restricted ambitions, imagination still dares to weave its way into their renditions, therefore reclaiming some of its vitality. A simple alteration in tone, theme, or timing can bring everything to life again. The voice seeks out the instrument and the instrument the voice. It may well be a patchwork but the lightness and originality of this little rhapsody combining the familiar with the different have their own charms. The game is on again and, with this, some part of life seems to be restored.

The two friends don't talk much; they don't mention their fear or pain: music is their only line of communication. There is one time, though, when Simon comes to sit next to Lise in the corridor. He's just been alone with Solal for a while because the child is too weak to get out of bed and play the piano today, so the two of them just chatted. Lise and Simon now sit in silence, side by side, looking at the closed piano.

"Do you know," Simon says, suddenly turning to Lise as if on an impulse, "I always knew I liked Solal, before. But not this much."

Lise doesn't reply. Nothing else of the sort will ever be said again. Lise and Simon will go on making music together for many years to come. Their friendship will grow, consolidated by these harmonies. Only once, four years later, will Simon mention the Institute to Lise again. Admitting how deeply affected he was by these months. Saying that he wasn't aware of it at the time. The visits didn't cost him anything then, but later, when it was all over, he had flashbacks, nightmares, *even dizzy spells. He often had painful memories of that hospital, of Solal and the other sick children. And it had an appreciable effect on his life. Lise won't be surprised to hear this. She always saw her friend's commitment if not as a sort of heroism, at least as recklessness. But then maybe that's what being a friend means.*

STOWAWAYS

There's always an inside and an outside. A within and a without. Things, living beings, social entities, places, words—nothing escapes this law and yet these concepts are relative. It's all down to point of view: depending on the angle of observation, surface can become depth, appearance essence, and the strange familiar. The outside inside. Boundaries are constantly redefined. Endlessly movable.

Life at the Institute depends on this paradigm shift. Anyone who comes here must appropriate things that are fundamentally alien, and assimilate this new world, learning its customs and becoming familiar with its codes. In the early stages, newcomers tend to adopt the reflex responses of foreigners in a host nation, withdrawing into themselves and their families, ghettoizing themselves. But this retreat doesn't last: integration comes fast. They become acclimatized, accustomed, they gain autonomy. Within a few days they've settled. They are connected by a sort of collective identification. Hospitality transforms exile into integration. It may appear comforting, but this evolution has problems of its own, and *this is because these same people still have to keep revisiting the old world. Inhabiting two different spaces and moving in two distinct timescales, they feel they're living two lives. It's not easy splitting themselves in two like this. They soon feel torn between contradictory affiliations. At home they can't stop thinking about the Institute; at the Institute, about home.*

Prosaic it may be, but in many cases this proves to be a simple quantitative question. Whichever parent is still working spends less time at the hospital, or at least less waking time. He or she often visits only in the evenings, and sometimes at night. That's a lot in itself, for sure, but not enough to make the place feel like another home. Caught in an infernal triangulation between work, home, and the Institute, this parent is also permanently confronted with many difficulties. He or she spends restless nights on cots, takes hasty showers in the early hours, and has extra commuting to do. In spite of everything, though, these parents know where home is, and home remains their point of reference. By contrast, the other parents, those who've abandoned any social function, struggle with questions of identity. The fact that they are a part of this place but are simultaneously from somewhere else means, paradoxically, they are residents in neither. They feel stateless. Foreigners here, foreigners there, like the children of immigrants. And so they must endlessly reposition themselves, redefine their criteria, reevaluate what they say, and adapt how they behave in search of inclusion. The toing and froing is exhausting.

In this instance, lymphoma provides a solution of sorts. By needing the patients' mothers to be at the Institute virtually the whole time, it removes the time factor. It decides for them and dictates to them, forcibly giving them a residence visa. The world gradually recedes, and the refuge is substituted for home. Eventually there is a total reversal. The Institute becomes their only reference point, the basis around which the geometry of their daily lives is built. The usual order of things no longer exists; another logic has taken over. It is in fact a very peculiar phenomenon: all at once everything outside the hospital seems strange; what felt natural only yesterday is suddenly open to question. Normality seems eccentric; ordinary things are tinged with exoticism. When they leave the walls of the Institute, these parents behave like travelers lost in some faraway land with outlandish customs. The layout of the city, the plethora of streets, the institutions, the politics, the leisure activities, the conversations in bistros, the gossipmongers, the snappy dressers and the sassy dressers—everything's a source of amazement to them. They view their former peers with the startled bewilderment of an ancient Huron or Persian in Paris. At first they may draw some strength from this, influenced by a sense of irony combined with a longing still to be a part of that world, but they soon lose any appetite for it. They then willingly retreat to the Institute, weary of their foray into Absurdia and convinced that they're finally back where they belong.

———

A coffee three mornings a week, a very few dinners cooked by brave and devoted friends and family (a couscous one time, a fondue another, and oysters at Christmas), and a birthday supper in the spring. That's all. It's enough. And yet everyone's doing his or her best here: our friends to take our minds off things, and us to spare their feelings. But we're here and not here at the same time, because there's no question of discussing the one thing that preoccupies us the most. We sympathize about upset stomachs, head lice, problems at school, and squabbles. We harrumph about shameless bosses, unemployment, injustice, global warming, and wars. We comment on a news item that we haven't been following, refer to shows we haven't seen, and plan vacations we won't take. We celebrate good news, smile at witticisms, and laugh at jokes. We fool them all every time, still chatting in this ancient language that no longer feels entirely like our own. Ours is incommunicable, a language whispered in intimate moments. It's incomprehensible and cannot be interpreted. It's inaudible, too painful to hear. We'd rather keep it quiet. The only things that spring from it are our children's love and the strength that keeps us going.

Inhabitants of the Institute may rarely venture outside, but movement in the opposite direction proves equally limited. And that's because the place is fairly protectionist. Not just anyone gets to enter. Other than professionals, parents, and occasionally grandparents, right to entry is granted sparingly and depends on the wishes—and present condition—of the child patient. And these don't necessarily coincide. There's no free exchange, which is a good thing, to be honest. Applicants are fairly rare, anyway. A visit to the Curie constitutes a grueling journey that not many are prepared to undertake. A spirit of adventure holds no weight because the place is too disorienting. So there are few applications and therefore few refusals. But the outside world can come up with other means of entry: there are stowaways.

First of all there are telephones. A phone means you can be here without making the trip, therefore avoiding any problems associated with the journey. A connection can be nurtured like this, avoiding issues of hygiene, vulnerability, or appropriateness. It spares both visitor and resident from possible overload. Because they're not experienced physically, eye contact is less freighted, tears less heartbreaking, and distress more bearable. "Lise, I'm calling…"—silence, gulp, sob—"I'm calling to…"—silence, gulp, sob—"I'm calling to…"—silence, sighing, intake of breath—"oh, damn it, I'm calling to say… I don't know what to say." Lise laughs. "Well, there you go, that's a wonderful, supportive thing to say. And plus you made me laugh! I'm glad you called. Thanks." It's actually very easy. And it means a lot. There's nothing else to say. Still, some people can't even talk, afraid it's a bad time or they'll say one thing too many, but they want to be there so they show their solidarity by text. Voice substitutes for a person, and then the written word for a voice. Thousands of words infiltrate the Institute like this every week: thoughts, encouragement, kindnesses—like so many demonstrations of affection transmitted in abbreviations, archiphonemes, and emoticons. It's a private backslapping exercise: one friend texts Lise every day to tell her how strong she's being, another sends her smileys, hearts, and flowers once a week, a third regularly sends her weird pictures found on the internet. The child, meanwhile, spends a lot of time messaging his friends, godparents, and cousins. His cell phone, which he was given four years early because of his isolation for health reasons, now provides a condensation of his social life, is its kindly messenger. Every day mother and child wait for these words and images, these signs of another life that is still possible. This waiting fills and structures their time, conferring a human density on an elastic present.

It doesn't stop at phones. A good many outside objects manage to make their way through the Institute's frontiers. Trafficking is established, sneaking things past the illness like a smuggler. It uses the parents' apartment as a depot for fencing goods. In this intermediary space between the world of the well and the world of the sick, dozens of things are gathered with the hope of gaining access to the hospital ward. These things have a tremendous presence, like well-meaning ghosts haunting the place as they seek the missing child. They bring the apartment to life and banish solitude.

In the first instance, they're things in writing: get-well cards, posters, little notes that are collaged into walls of images and transported from room to room. Copies of classwork too, because every Saturday Solal's teacher outlines the work his class has done so that he can follow every step of the way. Then there are books, comics, mangas, and games. One of these assumes special importance: it was put together by a group of students' parents, friends of Lise and Olivier, so that they could be with Solal every day. It's a file folder with a planisphere on the cover along with a title: "Where is it? Who is it?" Every week Solal's parents receive a brown envelope containing a piece of paper with a photo of one of Solal's school friends disguised in the traditional dress of a country, and a short brain-teaser. Solal has to identify the country implied and the friend in disguise. It's like a spy mission and is, of course, a wonderful invitation for his imagination to travel. Not only because it means his thoughts can escape to Canada, China, Hawaii, Mongolia, Lapland, or Egypt, but also because these geographical enigmas are like so many fragments of free poetry filled with the inventiveness of childhood. They're written in prose, in verse, in Morse code; presented as rebuses, riddles, and fairy tales; and combine letters, numerals, and images. Carried by this content, Solal visits the land of beavers, skunks, and caribou, travels across the country of compasses, paper, and gunpowder, explores the island where they eat lilikoi *and celebrate* Banana Poka, *meets the nation of horsemen where eagles are princes, skims the Arctic*

Circle with its brightly colored auroras, and ventures down into tombs where kings sleep for all eternity. He sets off on an adventure every week, enticed by the combination of discovery, expectation, and challenge, turning successive pages that always eventually bring him back to something so close to home, something familiar, a friend. "Where is it? Who is it?" Simple questions that—thankfully—replace other, unresolvable ones, so this game populates the empty hours and the dull downtime.

It's not only Solal's mind that feeds on these faraway places—the family's friends have also decided to sustain them bodily. They regularly bring the parents dishes from all over the world, preparing specialties from countries they've visited or that they come from. Their offerings include Italian risotto, Algerian couscous, Brittany pancakes, a Parisian epiphany cake, Japanese sushi, Chinese dumplings, Belgian waffles, and even termites from Cameroon. A real gastronomic round-the-world trip. If the cook is of a literary bent, he or she accentuates the migratory intensions, making the metaphor clear. Lise receives this text from one friend: "Norwegian immigrant seeks fridge space with the Ms. Immediate delivery available. Please get in touch." She replies: "Immigrant very welcome, no passport required." It turns out to be a particularly delicious salmon.

Words, things, and food offer some permanence in this break from the real world. They are talismans, snippets of eternity subsumed from whatever the future has in store. Like

the little bonsai that a friend leaves outside their door one day.
All these things remind Lise of the "inestimable present" that
Jean Tardieu refers to in a poem she once set to music. They
endow "what belongs to no one" with "intimacy amidst chaos,"
the "long wait" that brings together those who love each other,
"the unsaid things in their words" and "their shared but separate dreams." More than anything else, though, they offer "the
boundlessness of time at the very heart of a fleeting moment."

There's always an outside and an inside. A within and a without. Nothing can get away from that. Which is why there are
frequent stowaways, secret bearers of happiness, crossing borders and connecting different people and different worlds.

TO THE MOON

I'm a war machine. A force advancing toward and against everything. I never stop. I carve through the air and will keep going till the bitter end.

I'm at the Institute. I found my place here and no longer question my identity, my origins, my legitimacy, or my abilities. What I am, where I'm from, where I'm going—it all feels obvious. I've stopped hesitating; I know precisely, I just know. And, at last, I have the nerve.

I am Marie Curie. I reverently follow in the footsteps of Maria Salomea Skłodowska, sensing within me the ordinary continuation of her woman's genius, like a modest inheritance to remote descendants. Maternal devotion is my little laboratory, my lecturer's stool, my Nobel shadow. I work there every day, developing my secret research and my futile fight against cancer. I am just one thing: cure. *Cura*, care, concern, healing.

I'm yours. You're my religion, my creed, my vocation. I live off the love I have for you. It rouses me and sustains me, spurs me on and galvanizes me. The air I breathe is the hope of curing you. I can resist thanks to your resistance.

I exist thanks to your very existence. Self-abnegation is my brand of selfishness and my source of pride. I sacrifice myself to what is most essential to me.

Lise has stopped believing in God. Did she ever believe in him? At least now she dares come clean and say so. This ultimate blow of fate has gotten the better of her agnosticism. She'd forged herself a substitute for faith in the form of a gamble: if by any chance there was some sort of god, it would be a shame to upset him, to miss out on eternity for such a small thing, so she made a point of remaining undecided. As a precaution, mostly. She's through with that now. A being capable of inflicting so much infamy on childhood doesn't deserve respect. The logic of her gamble collapsed in the face of his blind lack of justice. And so now Lise believes only in existence, even lived in its most repulsive absurdity. Still, she does sometimes need to address her prayers to someone.

She feels this need particularly acutely when she arrives home from the Institute one evening. She's standing on the balcony of the apartment, leaning on the railings, smoking away her exhaustion. The smoke drifts off, coiling in the orangey light of the Paris sky. Lise hates this non-night in the city, this artificial distortion of the living world. She looks up: higher above she can in fact make out darkness and some stars. The moon is watching her. Full and complete, it extends over the

entire universe, like a whole note in a bar on the stave. It provides the scansion for passing time, sets a rhythm to the cycle
of people's lives, their mornings and evenings, their work and
their days. "That's who I can pray to," Lise thinks. "It'll do just
as well as a cipher with a white beard, and at least it chimes
with my love of nature. After all, the Greeks never stopped to
wonder whether they believed in their myths. The stories were
there because they were told, and that was enough." She then
remembers that a few years earlier Solal admitted to her that
he believed in all the gods of every religion, all together. When
she told him that ancient polytheism was a thing of the past,
he looked both surprised and disappointed. "You mean no one
believes in Poseidon anymore?" he asked. "No, honey, but
everyone does their own thing when it comes to faith. You have
every right to believe in him if you want to." Solal decided to
believe in Poseidon in spite of everything. And this evening,
Lise has decided to believe in the moon.

For a long time she simply stares at the moon in silence, as
if waiting for some sort of spiritual emanation. Then she talks
to it, in her head at first, then out loud, softly. She smiles as
she does it, feeling ridiculous, and a little crazy. Ridiculous
and a little crazy but still doing the right thing. In tune with
herself. First, she asks for a total and complete recovery for
her child. Not an improvement, not remission, but a full and
whole cure. An irreversible one. It's a lot to ask, she realizes
that, so in return she makes a promise, a commitment: she
swears to the moon that if her son comes out alive, then she,

Lise, will explore the strange energy sustaining her through this fight. And more significantly she'll explore the absence of this energy in other, more straightforward situations. She will ask herself why she has only ever been fired up with drive and strength for other people. Why she's always had to listen, help, entertain, and endure. Why she hasn't truly started to exist in her own eyes. She swears that, with her son saved, she will do for herself what she's currently doing for him. She'll work toward being reborn. Someday, after Curie, she'll take care of herself. If and only if the moon consents to save her son.

BALD 1

It's a slow, assured, expansive gesture. With its fingers held together the hand folds in on itself slightly to form a small hollow in the middle of the palm. First, it strokes the child's head, following the curve of his skull. It hardly seems to be in contact with his hair but appears instead to hover just above it. Perhaps it's just touching tiny little hairs barely visible to the naked eye. All the same, the child must be able to feel the hand, because every time it passes over him his closed eyes smooth out and his eyebrows arch. It actually makes for a very strange picture: this delicate skimming action by such a uniquely large, firm hand. Particularly as the gesture doesn't stop there. Once over the rise of the skull, the hand lingers for a moment in the vale below, on the hillside at the nape of the neck, before climbing back up toward the shoulder. It picked up a suggestion of speed on the way down, gaining some momentum that allows it to tackle the rise of the clavicle with serenity. Here again the movement is smooth and supple. It seems it might continue indefinitely, following the undulations of the child's body and tracing a soft sine curve in the air. But it doesn't. Once it reaches the point of the acromion the *hand does not embrace the outer curve of the shoulder; instead it continues to rise in a straight line and completes its arc much higher, almost twenty inches from the shoulder. Then it embarks on a transverse trajectory, as if hesitating before dropping back down. It couldn't really be called a turn, more a slight inclination, but, if watched closely, the hand can be seen to descend gradually toward a more distant point. And it continues like this, drawing its growing, expanding sinusoid. A whole yard away, at the end of a now outstretched arm, the hand appears to have reached its goal at last. It comes to rest peacefully, opens and spreads itself flat over a gray cardboard receptacle shaped like a bean. Or a kidney. Here it pauses. Then gently resumes its course, tracing a large loop in reverse, cutting through the air, and, without further interruptions, returning to its starting point on the child's hair. And then the whole thing starts again. Ten times, twenty times, the hand steadily and faithfully follows the same trajectory. In fact it becomes difficult to say whether it's the graceful movement itself, its assurance, or its identical iterations that produce such a soothing feeling. Unless this feeling is the result of the now perfect balance between strength and gentleness. Because this hand stroking, comforting, lulling, and mothering the sick child is large, powerful, and robust as a father's hand. A hypnotic sight. The viewer could willingly succumb indefinitely to its sinuous progress that reverses and turns on itself like a Möbius strip.*

After a few minutes, however, something seems to disturb the serene atmosphere. It's not immediately clear what. No incident has interrupted the harmony; the gesture still proceeds with the same regularity, in the same silence. Still calm, gentle, and assured—everything is unchanged. And yet there's an awkwardness, a sort of disturbing strangeness whose cause is difficult to identify. As if an intangible form has snuck into this intimate scene to disturb its familiar routine. And paradoxically the watcher's eye is drawn to this invisible presence. Imperceptibly, it abandons the hand to its movements and returns to the piece of cardboard where the hand came to rest moments earlier. The indefinable something seems to emanate from here. The eye changes its focus only slowly. It must be difficult to tear itself away from the fascination of this hand and its choreographic reiterations. But there's something else. It's as if the eye knows that it's heading toward a disturbing truth, something that should remain hidden. Unable to resist, it slows cautiously on its approach. Fear germinates and grows with the imminence of this secret transgressed. When the eye finally alights on the cardboard bean, it is full of dread. It can now see the inside of the receptacle, stripped of the discreet cover afforded by the hand. Some indescribable thing has curled up inside, molded to the curve of the cardboard, spilling over its edges and swelling in the center. It's black, hairy, and fat. Impossible to tell whether it's alive. It doesn't appear to be breathing, but no one could swear to that. It could have breathed once, at any rate. It actually looks like a dead rat, deposited still warm in its supine position into its cardboard coffin. There's definitely something corpse-like about the thing. It's an arresting, horrifying sight, but the horror doesn't last because the hand, having finished its cycle, is on its way back. And along with it come the cause and meaning of the thing. Hidden in the hand's large palm are a few black hair-like threads that it deposits into the receptacle. They instantly blend with the thing, increasing its volume. The whole of it then settles and coalesces under the weight of the hand, so that when the hand starts its movement again the only discernable shape inside the bean is a single homogenous mass. It's not a structured organism, then, but just an accumulation of disparate components aggregated into an impression of corporeality. But the eye wasn't completely misled: what's piling up here is in fact a biological substance. Let's follow the palm's progress again; once it has released its contents it does in fact return to the source or, put more crudely, the loading station. And now it's easy to recognize in the child's hair the substance previously identified in the bean. That's what it is, unquestionably. Not a dead body, but hundreds of fragments of a dying tegumentary system. Withered human pili that the hand gathers, harvests, and collects with every stroke before removing them and stowing them in that rigid, inert coffin. And it's no small torment seeing such grace and tenderness jointly and tactfully evidencing decline.

When I arrive at the Institute that morning, you're lying on your side in bed, facing the door. Head tilted and legs bent at forty-five degrees, your body sketches a tentative S shape under the covers. It seems to have attempted to adopt a fetal position and wasn't able to for some reason. Perhaps because of the cardboard receptacle sitting on the bedcover in the crook of your knees. You wouldn't have dared curl your legs right up to your chest for fear of spilling its contents. Your father's hand lying flat on the thing as if to keep it in position seems to substantiate this hypothesis. You don't open your eyes when I come in. Your father, who's sitting on the far side of you on a level with your shoulders, looks at me sadly. Then he looks away, apparently concentrating on the movement of his hand, which arcs up from the crook of your knees to the top of your head. He strokes your hair and then his hand follows some invisible outline in the air before coming to rest on the cardboard bean again. After a brief pause, the movement is repeated identically, and continues tirelessly. The curve, the outline, the cardboard, the pause, the curve, the outline, the cardboard, the pause, the curve, the outline, the cardboard, the pause. At first I let the constancy and aestheticism of the gesture hypnotize me: the lean torso behind your horizontal body, the arm going back and forth in periodic undulations, like the mast of a boat with a flapping sail regularly skimming the deserted decks on the whims of the swell. I savor this momentary respite from torment. I'm glad that you have such a tender man, such a loving father by your side, and I can admire his firm, elegant, gentle hand. His pianist's hand.

All at once I shudder: now I see and now I understand. The black thing that this beautiful hand has just deposited isn't a fluffy little creature it was protecting, huddled in its cardboard nest. Nor is it unprepossessing vermin—a sewer rat, street cat, or prying mole—that the hand has put in this makeshift shelter out of pity. Nor even the corpse of some disgusting animal. And yet it is to do with both life and death. It's from you and it's dead. When I look at you again, you still have your eyes closed, but where your eyelids meet, between your eyelashes, tears are beading.

Your father and I knew that this time would come. In fact, we expected it sooner. It's just a week late. You knew about it too. It was your father who warned you early on in the treatment, one night when you couldn't sleep. I came along in the morning and it was done. You knew. I didn't take it well at first. Not that he was the one to have told you, but because he and I hadn't discussed it beforehand to decide on the right time and how to break the news. You cried a lot, apparently, and I wasn't there to console you. It was hard. That's what happened and, in the end, what does it matter? Is there really a time, a person, a choice of words, or a way of delivering this fact that's more appropriate than any other? It certainly wouldn't change anything for you. And anyway, the three of us had an opportunity to discuss it further that same morning. I was able to answer your questions, explain the reasons, and reassure you about the consequences. And most of all emphasize that this alopecia would be only temporary. Tell you that hair usually grows back glossier and softer as soon as the treatment is over. I was there to hold you close and try to soften the blow of this news and the harshness of the facts.

Today, though, words and reasons and reassurances prove powerless. What is there to say about this heartbreak and your outrage? Every stroke of your father's hand sweeps up hundreds of vestiges of your hair. Nearly a million follicles are emptying themselves of their cells. The roots, deprived of nutrients, tear out. The capillary covering of your body is coming away in handfuls. The whole thing falling into ruins, disintegrating. You're losing your carapace, your peel, your covering, your armor. The thing that protects you from the cold, the heat, and blows, and that constitutes a key characteristic of your physical identity. Your highest feature. Your roof. So what is there to say, other than nothing? I sit on the bed, put one hand gently on your hip, and bring the other up to stroke your cheek with one finger. And the three of us stay there like that in silence, huddled around your pain.

The bean is very soon full and needs emptying. I ask you what you'd like to do with the gathered hair. You say you want to keep it as a souvenir. From one of the nurses I get my hands on a plastic wallet sealed with a zipper and, like a medical examiner, I slip these remnants escaping from your body into it. They not only carry your genome, but also crystalize the memory of a before. Their desertion is a tangible sign of your illness. From root to tip, the fall of each individual hair is visible proof of the stealthy wreckage of your intimate being. It demonstrates the slow devastation of your cells, your violated, pillaged, ransacked cells abandoned inert to a sterile lifeless desert. Soon everyone—including us and you yourself—will see you as what lymphoma has made of you: a cancer patient. Soon your smooth, denuded scalp will scream for all to hear about your damaged body and heart. Soon you will be bald.

BALD 2

The child has run his right hand through his hair, gathered a fistful of it, and deposited it carefully into the open palm of his other hand. He's now intent on making it into a little bundle, rolling it between his thumb and index finger like dark tobacco. "What if we made a mustache with it?" His mother doesn't remember which of them came up with the idea, but it certainly appeals to them both. Especially as it's not difficult—an ordinary Band-Aid does the trick. When it's been rolled around the parcel of hair and then folded back on itself into a loop-shaped sticker, Lise positions it over her son's upper lip. The effect isn't bad if a little lopsided. The child looks in the bathroom mirror and plays up to it, screwing up his nose, winking an eye, twisting his mouth one way, then the other, alternately tilting up the two corners of the hairpiece. Bandy-legged and baggy-pajamaed, with his feet at ten to two and an imaginary walking stick in his hand, he makes a strange but happy Charlie Chaplin. But there's a missing accessory: he needs a bowler hat. His mother steals an avatar for this—a hygiene cap—from a cart left outside the nurses' room. "Your hat, *sir!" she says and the child laughs out loud. Small pleasures are worth a lot at the Institute.*

Viewed superficially, going bald actually is quite funny. It gives the person access to something extraordinary, reversing the course of time: at an age when everything should be grow- ing, time goes backward. And it accelerates too, as if every hair were hastily, in the space of just a few days, running through all the phases of its life cycle. Fifty of them should reach matu- rity every day, but now a hundred thousand of them die in one go. And lastly, time also stands still because once the shedding is over, no new follicles start to develop. It's quirky but also a little grotesque. Absurd. Besides, it offers opportunities to do things people never do: see the shape of their heads, and the color of them, and stroke their scalps. Tear their hair out, literally. Or do all sorts of things with it—cut bangs, put it in a French pleat, or a high ponytail, cut one particular lock out- rageously short, pull more hair from one side than the other, do it up like an Iroquois, a Rasta, a hedgehog, a lunatic, stiffen it into a punk's crest, braid the sparse tufts with beads and colored elastic like little African girls, cover the balding scalp with a straggly combover to look like old politicians on TV. Or all sorts of other recreational inventions. It doesn't matter. There won't be any left soon, anyway.

Solal has no lack of imagination in this field. He gets caught up in the game the very next day after the first loss. He's in the bathtub and has decided to wash his hair. There are already dozens of hairs floating on the surface of the water.

He pours some shampoo into his wet hand and lathers it over his head. When he takes his hand away the white foam is darkened by hundreds of hairs, fine threads diffracted by the bubbles. He looks up at his mother gleefully, "Look, Mommy. This is the only shampoo that can make your hair fall out!" "That would make a hell of a commercial," Lise replies. "Like the ones claiming they help hair grow back, but in reverse. Anyway, I can tell you, I've never been sure they don't cheat with their tests. If you ask me, they take a picture of a guy with plenty of hair and then shave it off. Then they switch the pictures and that's all there is to it. At least we're sticking to the right order." "What if we filmed a fake ad? Go on, Mommy, film me with your cell phone. Just my head, obviously." The child is suggesting a real parody here. He comes up with a name for the product, a jingle, a slogan, and a story-board, thrilled with his own inventions. Brandishing the bottle of shampoo, he triumphantly pulls out five successive handfuls of hair, proving how effective the product is. Then he reaches both arms to the ceiling in a victory V, flinging the bottle and the hair to opposite sides of the bathroom with a great roar of laughter, before throwing himself, soaking and giggling, into his mother's arms.

A few days later, at her son's request, Lise shows the video to a close friend. To her considerable surprise the friend doesn't find it funny; Lise is even aware of a sort of awkwardness. The friend has never seen Solal bald and is probably shocked, but there's something else: she doesn't seem to appreciate the little film's off-the-wall humor. The joke clearly isn't catching on, and this seems to be what's embarrassing her, as if the comedy were somehow misplaced. Lise now grasps something she didn't understand before: this laughter, that felt so natural to them, doesn't belong outside the Institute. It is peculiar to the circumstances. It isn't black humor or forced laughter, but a type of laughter all its own. It isn't ugly, sarcastic, or dark. It has no target and is intended only to be defensive. It's a laugh that bubbles up when everything is beyond control and nothing has any meaning anymore. It holds Lise and her son together, saving them from the unspeakable. It could easily become convulsive, hysterical even, but nevertheless guarantees a degree of sanity. It's the laughter of survival, incommunicable and for them alone.

PROSOPAGNOSIA

By the beginning of the second month I no longer recognize you. It happens suddenly with no warning. I'm sitting facing you one day, looking at you, talking to you, listening to you, and all at once I realize I don't recognize you. You've stopped corresponding to my sensory memory. Obviously, I know in my heart, my soul, and my mind that you're my son but there no longer seems to be anything—no sign, no physical or mental characteristic—by which I can identify you.

First of all there's your bald head. Or nearly bald, which is worse. Because here and there across the hairless expanses there are still islets of growth. Sometimes spiky and upstanding, sometimes flopping over as if stuck to your smooth skin. The hairs are dull and brittle; they look lank and weak, and seem to have huddled into little clusters of ten or twelve to wage one final battle against the enemy besieging them. It's Fort Alamo or the last of the Mohicans on your deserted scalp. To be honest, I'd prefer you to be completely bald: you'd still be you, but you'd have assumed your cancer patient head. The kind we all know because we've seen it on TV, on posters, in magazines, or in letters appealing for donations, usually alongside some media personality. The kind of head whose image has been skillfully reworked to make the illness seem both moving and familiar, sad and beautiful. A half smile, a diaphanous complexion, luminous eyes, a smooth, polished, rounded scalp, just a few injunctions to hope. A shrewd disposition to frighten people, but not too much, so that they can view it with a carefully calibrated combination of empathy, fear that they may themselves be affected someday, and relief that they aren't right now—all reactions likely to trigger the act of giving. But the little clumps of sparse hair on your head don't tally with these aesthetic representations of cancer. This half measure is ugly, distressing, and faintly ridiculous. You wouldn't reap a single cent, that's for sure. It doesn't look like anything recognizable. Or rather it does, come to think of it, you remind me of Gollum, the repulsive creature invented by Tolkien: pale, withered, with huge, avid eyes and scattered stringy hairs over an ovoid head. A corrupt individual who's both endearing and threatening. A monster produced by the metamorphosis of a hobbit.

It's not just your hair; everything's changed. Your face, with cheeks swollen by cortisone, is a drab color between beige and grayish brown. Your muscles have melted away and you look puny. Your smell has changed too: you smell of vomit, mouthwash, and antiseptics. You smell of the hospital, you don't smell of you anymore. Your voice is unrecognizable too, it's grown higher as it's become quieter. It's now reduced to a reedy thread of barely articulated sounds. No sentences, no words even, just rambling disjointed monosyllables that make no sense. Besides, you've stopped trying to communicate. You moan in a constant stream of little cries, like the stifled mewling of a newborn. You also struggle to move around; this deformed body doesn't obey you properly. You can take only small steps now, slowly sliding your feet over the floor one after the other, as if they've become too heavy to lift. You talk like a baby but you walk like an old man, concatenating the two extremes of life in their all-encompassing weakness, but failing to reconcile them harmoniously. It's unbearable to behold. And this is the source of the horror: not so much the ugliness in itself but the feeling of suddenly being confronted with the image, crystallized in this frail individual, of the full extent of the human condition held in the vise that crushes it between two oblivions. That's what your treatment has made of you: a hybrid creature that goes against nature, a terrifying mixture of regression and senescence, tottering on the edge of the abyss, so ready to return to the non-being from which it has only just emerged.

This deterioration could be limited to your physical appearance, but your spirit seems to have collapsed too. It's left you with a gaping black hole inside you. You're naturally so luminous but you now radiate only gloom. Where have all the hopes gone, the rages, tears, dreams, and childish joys that still managed to surface up until now? You don't want anything anymore, you don't hope for anything and don't reject anything. You seem to have stopped fighting. I'm so afraid you're giving up. Only yesterday you were still laughing but I can't get you to sketch the rudiments of a smile today. Yesterday you still described your pain but I can't get you to talk today. The truth is, I can't even establish contact with you. You've shut yourself away in repetitive stereotypical gestures: your fingers twisting and clutching at each other, fretfully contorting a piece of fabric—a T-shirt or a sheet; giving off little bleats at irregular intervals; drifting slowly and aimlessly backward and forward in the corridor. As with autistic conditions, the behaviors preclude any attempt at interaction. Lymphoma has taken possession of you. I've lost you.

I'm ashamed to say it but I'm frightened and repelled by the new face that is now yours. I don't try to understand this feeling of otherness, I just hate myself for feeling it. How can a mother lose all conviction of her son's identity like this? I recognized you when you were born, even before I knew what you would look like and who you would be. Our connection isn't based on familiarity, so how can it be threatened by some internal or external transformation? And how can this affect my intuition of your belonging? Could I bring you back into the world anonymously now on the grounds that you're not the same anymore? The thought horrifies me. I'm losing my mind. Maybe

I'm scared that I'll give up too, that I won't know how to keep going, that I won't be able to keep supporting, helping, and loving you properly. That I'll abandon you. And what if I'm wrong? What if it's actually me who's sick? A failing in my cerebral processes, a cognitive malfunction, a sudden perceptual blindness that means I can no longer identify you. Something like prosopagnosia but going beyond mere visual damage and spreading to the other senses. That's it, I get it: I have a generalized condition that means I don't recognize familiar faces, voices, smells, and tastes. The sensory information is empty and inadequate. I have total agnosia. Perhaps the trauma triggered the symptoms. Unless, conversely, they've developed specifically to protect me. Because of course it would suit me just fine for you not to be my son. For this pained, defeated creature teetering on the edge to be someone else. For my Solal to be somewhere different, safe and sound. Maybe that's also why you've chosen to disappear, burying yourself into your impenetrable depths, the better to escape the abomination. Confronted with cruel reality, you've taken refuge in your deepest fortress, carefully locking every exit. And there, safe and warm, you'll wait. If you're not found, you can't be caught. Like an organism battling hypothermia, its blood retreating from its limbs to fill the vital organs. And what if this were the chrysalis that you wished for in the early days of your treatment? Not the nymph's intermediary stage, its metamorphosis, but the protective envelope of a creature in the making. It just hasn't adopted the expected form. We pictured a fine, delicate membrane, something transparent or at least translucid, a soft, welcoming cocoon. So naturally we're surprised to find something grotesque and repulsive instead. But this is only a chimera, after all, a monstrous outward appearance protecting your inner self. Beneath this envelope of decrepitude, darkness, and silence, the essential you remains intact. You live on. I know you're still there, nestled in the dark. I mustn't force you out into the world but must respect your withdrawal and adopt your absence. This wall surrounding and protecting you may be off-putting but I shall surround and protect it in turn. My arms will act as an extra rampart so you can retreat still deeper inside yourself and hunker down there in secret. I will hug you close, your whole circumference.

When I finally put my arms around you, sensations return: my body remembers you by touch. You're the same boy I could already sense ten years ago, even though I'd never seen him. The same boy I carried within me and outside me. I recognize you. You're my child.

BALD 3

I t's a slow, intent, meticulous gesture. The hand is tensed, grasping the tool. Its tendons bulge at the joints, and the last section of the index finger, which is bent back against a stop on the handle, has gone bright red all around the nail. The hand appears to be shaking slightly. Nevertheless, it traces a perfectly straight path over the child's head, about two inches wide and eight inches long. From a purely artistic perspective, it's a fairly remarkable sight. Between peaks of white foam, the strip of bared skin, gleaming with a combination of water and lubricating cream, emerges smooth and polished. It looks like a shining road revealed between two snowdrifts by a passing snowplow. The hand rinses the tool in a glass of warm water and then goes calmly back to its clearing work, stripping another path parallel to the first, from forehead to occiput. The gesture is repeated, imperturbable.

When and why did Lise decide to shave her son's head? She couldn't say precisely. She just remembers that his hair loss, which came later than expected, was as speedy as it was imperfect. In the space of forty-eight hours the child was almost bald, keeping only a few meager strands here and there.

Then nothing else happened, as if the hairs that had resisted the first damage, sickly though they looked, refused to give in. Everyone was secretly waiting for them to fall out. To no avail. Paradoxically, this partial survival was more of a blow to the mother than the alopecia proper, which she had accepted as a necessity, like proof of how tough, and therefore how effective, the treatment was. A hairless head testified to the possibility of victory. On the other hand, these pathetic, straggly remnants of hair demonstrated the whole process of decline and, along with it, the full extent of the risks. It made Lise's son look as if he were dying, and she found this unendurable. There was even apparently a point when she was afraid she'd never find the real Solal again. And so, bizarrely, the tenacity of these few hairs produces a feeling of loss. Better to make a clean sweep of it then. The idea became chiefly an aesthetic concern in Lise's mind. Despicable it may be, but a mother's subtle disgust probably remains more acceptable than the raw fear of death. So in the first instance the mother simply told herself that this patchy scalp was ugly and looked dirty. Then she thought how like an old man it made her son look. Lastly, she went so far as to admit to herself that she thought the child looked monstrous and she was really struggling to recognize him. At each of these stages, she felt the shadow of mortality hovering over her imaginings. But the question of appearance kept prevailing, saving her from descending into frantic anxiety. And so she willingly allowed herself to be won over by this obsession with a smooth, pristine naked scalp. She saw it as a white page, a blank canvas onto which the sterilized image of the perfect cancer could be projected. A cancer that would return the child to his or her indigenous beauty. A slick, hygienic, almost healthy sort of cancer. An absolutist logic was therefore established, and it drove Lise's decisions. This was about taking back control of their fate by following through the debilitating process undertaken by the chemotherapy and sublimating it into beauty. Literally perfecting hair loss and raising it to splendor. The plan is over-the-top. It's intrusive, nurtured by an illusion of ascendancy and control. It also most likely comprises an element of madness in response to the sheer absurdity of the situation. But the mother doesn't realize this; she leaves it at hoping that her son won't look so sick when it's done.

When it comes to the time, Lise regrets her initiative: her hand shakes as she picks up the razor, then hovers over his head for a moment, hesitating. And yet it all started so well. They talked about it and the child agreed to it; he was almost curious about the result. He too loathed the relics of hair that he claimed made him look like a mad scientist. He liked the idea of getting rid of them, almost found it funny. He and his mother turned it into a sort of playful challenge. They'd opted for a day when the child was at home, feeling relatively well between two courses of chemotherapy, to take action. They happily ran through the preparatory scene-setting process, transforming the living room into a barbershop: putting a first stool by the window as the "customer's" chair, then a second as a table for implements, and then setting out a glass of warm water, a clean cloth, and a razor on this second stool. The choice of tool was easy: the father's electric shaver wouldn't be appropriate if they were to achieve the necessary smoothness. The way its blades worked, hidden behind the fine foil head and not directly in contact with the skin, would be too approximative, and there was a rigidity to it that seemed incompatible with the curve of the child's head. Besides, the mother was afraid she didn't really know how to use it. It was likely to take several attempts, irritating what was already fragile skin. In fact, she felt that only her own simple razor, with its lubricating strips and ergonomic handle and designed to follow a woman's curves, could guarantee the right combination of protection and precision, suppleness and thoroughness. She was convinced that its open blades would be more delicate and sensitive. After all, hadn't various product managers—converted semiologists and other inspired creative types—given this modest implement the glorious name "Venus"? Solal definitely had nothing to fear under the aegis of this goddess. To be extra safe, though, Lise had chosen to use it in combination with shaving foam. She didn't usually use foam but found a forgotten can of it in a drawer. Not knowing where it was from or how old it was, mother and son laughed a lot as they pictured the skin reactions that might result from using a product past its expiration date—blisters, hives, spots, pustules, boils, and bubonic lesions. They particularly enjoyed inventorying these diverse monstrosities, labeling them like jars of formaldehyde containing shapeless creatures lined up on the shelves of some cabinet of curiosities or museum of anatomy. This madcap teratology diverted tragedy into a farcical melodrama, and it helped them picture the ordeal and ready themselves for it. Added to this was the application of the aforementioned foam to the almost bare scalp—a process with a flavor all its own. It looked like whipped cream heaped onto a perfectly plump golden choux pastry, but utterly indigestible. At the same time, however, they couldn't help noticing the irony of the situation; the foam gave the child an artificial head of hair precisely when he was to be stripped completely bald. For now at least he had no need for a wig. Satisfied with his new face, the child stepped down from his stool to go admire himself in the mirror, posturing as some grand figure from the Ancien Régime, a king, nobleman, or court musician. That was still kind of fun.

And yet, in spite of everything, Lise is hesitating now. She's frightened of hurting the child. He probably guesses this misgiving and asks whether she's sure about what she's doing. She says yes, of course she is, she knows what she's doing. She's not used to lying to him, this may be the first time she's allowed herself to since his lymphoma started. Granted, she's occasionally omitted details or held back disturbing facts, but she's never openly distorted the truth like this. Still, how could she admit to her son that she's terrified at the thought of cutting him, while also unsure she can avoid doing it? It's too late to backtrack so she just tries to calm the shaking in her hands and her heart's anarchic beating. Then she wets the razor in *the warm water and traces the first track, swiftly followed by two more, without a hitch. Nevertheless, the action becomes more complicated when she needs to skirt around his ears and reach the temporal and occipital areas. A bit of vigilance is needed now. There are curves, projections, and angles, and tracing out straight lines is no longer enough. Farther down below the occiput, the twin outlines of the trapezius muscles create a valley inside which, forming another crest, is the top of the cervical vertebrae. All these escarpments are like obstacles where the razor could catch and tear the skin. Wounds must be avoided at all costs; the child will be in complete aplasia in a few days so this is definitely no time to breach his cutaneous barrier and offer infectious agents an entry point into his organism. The mother therefore proceeds slowly, calmly, and cautiously. The blades glide and skim over Solal's head rather than touching it. It's unusual to see a cutting instrument perform such a tender movement—shaving with all the gentleness of a mother's caress.*

The result is beyond satisfactory: Once the child's scalp is rinsed and massaged with soothing cream, it looks smooth and almost satiny. It's perfect. In his mother's opinion, the boy's no longer simply beautiful but glorious. The absence of hair accentuates the almond shape of his dark eyes. Combined with the clean, regular lines of his mouth, nose, and chin, and with his bronze skin, it lends him an air of refined distinction. With his graceful hands and upright head carriage, he looks like an Asian prince, although it wouldn't be easy to say where he's from because his face now goes beyond his acknowledged Judeo-Tunisian ancestry and suggests more far-flung places. There's something Egyptian, Slavic, and even Kazakh in this child but that's nothing new—Solal is simply reviving a unique quality he already had as a baby but that faded with time. Lise remembers that when she took her son out in his stroller people often asked her whether he was Eurasian mixed race. She liked it, not so much for the subsequent aesthetic compliments they paid but for the multicultural horizons it opened. The boy's beauty seemed to be living testimony of a fertile and flamboyant history, extrapolating the real adventures of his paternal line. It simultaneously endorsed the trials and courage of exiles, the vigor of his origins, the cultural wealth of mixing races, the lasting nature of memory, and the energy of new beginnings. This wasn't simply about the way Solal's ancestors were scattered about the Middle East, North Africa, and southern Europe; the beauty of this firstborn son single-handedly summarized every diaspora. It established the mysterious land of family legend that had been reinvented by the boy's young parents. A lot for a baby to shoulder. And yet, fictional though it was, this narrative means that Lise recognizes her child today. And to achieve that she still needs the intermediary of a face completely alien to his ancestry. Solal is bald and looks like a bald person . . . but not just any old bald guy. He has the distinctive elegance of a Yul Brynner, an actor able to incarnate the King of Siam, Ramses II, a sultan, a mercenary, General Bounine, and Dimitri Karamazov.

An actor of mixed origins that were deliberately kept secret and imprecise—Russian, Jewish, Romany, Swiss, or Mongolian. A majestic, inscrutable man committed to making a complex myth of his own life. And it's paradoxically this other man, this screen figure, this self-mythologizer whom Solal has never heard of and who isn't a member of his family, this man who was mysterious about his origins, which he may not even have known himself, it's this man—because he is both bald and glorious—who restores the child's identity and brings him back to his mother.

Lise gazes at her son, full of emotion. She kisses him and says, "You're gorgeous. You look like Yul Brynner." His almond eyes open wide, unconvinced.

"Who's Yul Brynner?"

YOUR BODY IS
NO LONGER YOUR BODY

Your body's no longer yours. It doesn't belong to you anymore. It belongs to all the people who look at you, assess you, examine you, feel you, measure you, weigh you, lay you down, get you up, sit you down, put you on a bed, disinfect you, inject you, remove needles from you and put needles back into you; those who wash you, feed you, hydrate you, and tend to you; even those who soothe you, stroke you, massage you, comfort you, hug you, and cuddle you. It also belongs to the port-a-cath that has penetrated it and can be seen in the protuberance under your skin, to the metal needle linking the inside to the outside of you, to the plastic tube that seems to spring from your collarbone like a hideous excrescence, to the multiple tentacles that grow out of it along its length, and even to the drip pole where these same limbs come together to hang from different-colored pouches. And lastly it belongs to the molecules that bombard you on the inside, destroying your cells, dulling your skin, swelling your face, thinning your limbs, slowing your growth, and making your hair fall out. Deformed, distorted, wilted. Alien.

Your body's no longer yours. It's completely given over to suffering and to sickness. It belongs to lymphoma.

Fight. Breathe out, breathe in, listen, feel, dream, play, draw, read, sing, dance, sleep, laugh, cry, scream, walk away. Feel this body in every way. Reclaim it from them, from all these people. Reclaim it from us. It's yours. It belongs to you.

EULOGY

Don't you sometimes think you'd rather have a different little boy instead of me? A kid who's not sick. Who's not in danger of..."

I don't know what hurts me most in these words: the doubt you imagine in me; the third conditional and its possible horizons; or that final ellipsis, where you leave your life dangling. No, Solal, I don't think that. I've never thought it. I don't want another child instead of you, whatever the situation. I can put your mind at rest about that right away.

On the other hand, I can't get to sleep that night. My mind has held on to the words, they've opened a painful fissure. For months now we've been moving forward along a tightrope over the void, pretending to ignore the abyss at our feet. Sometimes a breath of air makes us wobble, a fever that won't go down, a period of aplasia that goes on and on, a few days' delay in the protocol. We feel the draft from the wing of death breathe over us. It makes us shudder. At times like this the tightrope sways alarmingly. We slow down, clinging to our balancing poles, maintaining equilibrium. Whatever we do we mustn't look at our feet. We need to stare at a point up ahead, make out the other side of the chasm away in the distance.

But tonight I do need to cast an eye into the depths, to sound the abyss and surrender to the absurd. I'm committed to this by my insomnia, which produces periods of hypervigilance when my mind gets carried away and just takes me along in spite of myself. Thanks to insomnia, the uncertainty and the silence and the "if" that you planted in me grow. I chase after them, catch up with them, and soon overtake them. My thoughts race, an inextricable mixture of images and words spilling in every direction, branching and proliferating. I head off down different pathways, the pasts and the futures, the well-trodden and the untouched, the major routes and the byways. I write the imaginary novel of the worst that could happen and finally reach the last chapter.

We've come to the day of your death. Your body's lying in a white coffin and I'm standing behind a pulpit reading your eulogy. I have so much to say about this life that was yours, so much intimacy, so much tenderness, so much laughter, so much love and happiness. It's both terrifying and soothing. I've been down to the very depths, to the bitter end, and I now know that, whatever happens, I'll have it in me to thank you for sharing these ten years with us.

A FUNERAL

Your grandfather died last night. You're in the hospital undergoing chemotherapy and he's in the morgue. We'll have to tell you soon. A part of him already left us fourteen years ago; an accident made him a different person: problems with language, memory, and attention span; a combination of disinhibition and lack of interest; a sort of absent presence. Still a presence, though. But this time he's really gone, and it's cancer that took him.

On July 4, 1999, at the exact time when Olivier and Lise were exchanging their marriage vows at the Mairie in the Thirteenth Arrondissement of Paris, the groom's father, Jacques, known as Jacky, then sixty years old, electrocuted himself beside his swimming pool in the hills behind Cannes. Paris and Pégomas. The dream and the disaster. Life and death, already. Two dimensions that were discordant, contradictory, incompatible even, collided. It could almost have been seen as a sign of some cosmic disturbance: a universe in free fall, a sidereal storm, flashes of light streaking across space, roaring thunder, electromagnetic hurricanes, then two portals of fire, two phantasmagorical apertures opening in separate places, one on the waxed parquet floor of the Mairie, a peculiar extravagance amid its republican austerity, the other on the calm waters of the swimming pool, diffracting the light bouncing off it in a bizarre mise en abyme. But in truth there was none of this. Not a whisper, not a tremor. Each event progressed independently, unperturbed, conforming to its own logic, such a shocking concatenation of beatitude and catastrophe that it occurred in silence, in all the secrecy of cowardice.

Emotional and nervous, supported by close friends and family, the couple climbed the formal staircase, all blue carpet over stone steps, that led up to the marriage hall. Alone, in love and sunkissed, Jacky and Thérèse set off down the steps that snaked between the mimosas, palm trees, thyme, and oregano, breathing the warm air of a garden that dropped in a series of terraces to the swimming pool below. Olivier was wearing pale jeans and a brown linen jacket with a Mandarin collar, Lise a sandy-colored dress, also in linen. It was her favorite dress, she wore it a lot. Only a few accessories emphasized how special the occasion was, a delicate crocheted hat, hastily bought that same morning, and cream shoes, a discreet indication of the big family ceremony planned for the following week. Thérèse and Jacky took off their clothes. They would go naked, which is how they liked to be, exposing their ageing bodies on the warmed paving stones, naked in the suffocating *southern air, naked among the bees and bumblebees, the lavender, myrtle, and agapanthuses. Lise and Olivier drew closer to the two red velvet chairs intended for the bride and groom, the deputy mayor stood behind a desk under a photograph of the president, and their friends found seats behind them amid a restrained hubbub. Thérèse covered herself with sun cream and Jacky took a pressure washer from the tool shed. The deputy mayor gave his speech, reminding the couple of the nature of the commitment they were making and then, at last, pronouncing the ritual words. Thérèse took out a book, Jacky plugged the pressure washer into the extension lead.*

Thunderous applause, the couple hold hands, wave to their friends, and kiss each other. Lightning flash of the short-circuit. Jacky collapses, lifeless. Neurological crash, respiratory paralysis, cardiac arrest. Thérèse screams. Her husband's dying. Lying peacefully in the sun with his mouth open, he looks as if he's sleeping. But he is dying. He has two charred black holes, one on his right thumb, the other on his left heel.

Jacques didn't die on July 4, 1999. A neighbor, alerted by Thérèse's screams, came and administered first aid: heart massage and mouth-to-mouth resuscitation saved his life— and part of his brain—until the emergency services arrived ten minutes later. He stayed in a coma for more than a month and emerged from it distraught, incoherent, and wracked by involuntary movements. The initial prognosis was bleak and his physiotherapy protracted. He lost his job, his autonomy, his drive, his short-term memory, his brilliance, and his social and emotional attachments, but he did regain his vital functions. He recovered, although not fully, his mobility, the power of speech, and part of his memory. He still had his wife and family, and even recognized them eventually. Lise and Olivier canceled the big wedding party planned in a chateau in the Beaujolais region the following week. They didn't go on a honeymoon, choosing instead to go to his unconscious father's bedside every day that summer in the hope of bringing him back to the world with the sheer power of words, affection, and their presence. They stayed for hours at a time sitting at the hospital, looking out for signs—a blink, the twitch of a finger, a change in breathing—and lulled by the regular rhythm of the pump on the life support respirator. Two years later, during a post-coma checkup, Jacky was found to have stomach cancer. In time. In a way, his accident saved his life. His stomach was removed and the cancer then attacked his gallbladder. Then his peritoneum. The courses of chemo kept coming, the cancer kept metastasizing, his condition kept deteriorating, but Jacky kept going. "I'm rustproof," he liked to say. At least he hadn't lost his sense of humor. But he was really no more rustproof than anyone else. The cancer was eating away at him like a slow corrosion, gradually destroying his healthy organs, weakening his resilience, and diminishing his life. His decline was visible, the outcome in no doubt. They just didn't know when it would happen.

———

February 23, 2013. Your grandfather died of cancer last night. You too could die of it. Of course it's not the same thing, not the same illness. Who's going to be scared of a simple homonymy? But still. It's a painful coincidence. It has to be said, your grandfather definitely has a way with timing. The telephone rang at 3 a.m. and, woken with a start, our bodies reverberated to its terrifying echo for a long time afterward. You were at the Institute, alone, so far away from us, so fragile and vulnerable. Anything could happen to you. Your father picked up. Dare I say he was relieved when he heard his mother's voice? We knew what this meant, though. But most of all we knew what it didn't mean. And that was what mattered. Your father went straight to Gustave Roussy hospital, the other major oncology center. He came home early in the morning; Jacky was still holding out and they managed to talk to each other. To say goodbye. His last words before he sank into unconsciousness were about you. Your grandmother called back a little later. This time it was over. I don't know how your father got through those few extraordinary hours, my mind's struggling just to make sense of them. Losing his father when his son was on the brink. How does anyone deal with that? What sensations did he experience, what emotions bombarded his heart? Could he even grasp what was happening to him? I think that, in order to keep going, he must have partially closed himself off to this new pain. He barricaded himself in there, in the saddest place he could be, walling up his gaps, plugging his cracks, leaving his grief on the doorstep. There wasn't room for any more pain inside him.

This Saturday morning Lise has a specific task: picking up Solal from the Institute. His week of chemotherapy is coming to an end and he can come home for a few days until the next bout of fever that will see him rushed back to the hospital. As usual. But today will be different, she'll have to wait and pretend: wait for Olivier to come home so that, once the whole family is together, they can tell the children that their grandfather is dead; and in the meantime pretend everything's normal, betray nothing of the night's events, of the heartbreak and terrible dejection. Battle through this ordeal. Perhaps even compensate in anticipation of the predicted grief with an extra dose of cheerfulness. That shouldn't be difficult, really, with Solal coming home. Surely that's good cause for celebration in itself? When he gets home this afternoon they'll make pancakes.

In the end, it's not that simple, because this isn't to do with Lise disguising her current sorrow but with managing her husband's and children's sorrow to come. Yet again, she's not first in line, her pain is secondary. She's mostly suffering on other people's behalf. It's unbearable for her to think of Olivier crushed in the vise of this double agony, but harder still to know she must inflict it on her children. To be the messenger of this sorrow this evening, to be yet again and in such already difficult circumstances the bearer of bad news that is a strange echo of what is playing out. As if Jacky's death were suddenly giving substance to a buried, unspoken, unvoiced fear. An absolute fear. Solal's death. Lise wishes she could change time, erase the night's events, put them off till later, abolishing this abominable synchronicity, this irony of fate. That's impossible in real life so she must tackle this with her wits, building a watertight wall between the actual death and the dreaded one, to avoid any contamination of the one by the other. She must juggle any temptation to analogize. Must distinguish, separate, dissociate. All things considered, Lise decides that the best way to spare her children is not to ignore grief but instead to embrace it. It's only by fully experiencing this pain, by acknowledging this bruising absence, the bitterness of missing their grandfather and weeping for him, that the children will avoid the macabre coincidence. But they need to be told this evening.

The day passes happily, then the long-awaited moment comes. Everything seems perfectly normal; in other words, as it would be in any other family. The parents sit down with their children, trying to be both reassuring and concerned. The news is given in clear words and with tender gestures. Some tears flow, others are held back. Some questions are resolved, others cannot be answered. The family talks about Jacky, Thérèse, where they were from, where they met, how much they loved each other. Everyone contributes his or her own memories. A few photos are brought out. The children think of various friends who've also lost a grandparent. Paradoxically, this grief is a source of hope. They may not understand it, but it can be shared with others. There's something almost soothing about fitting in with the natural order of things like this, feeling like everyone else. It wouldn't take much for them to forget the lymphoma. Well, not that much. If Nils didn't ask why they were so unlucky. If Anna wasn't willfully holding back her pain. If Solal hadn't guessed straightaway, before his parents even opened their mouths. If the outline of the hideous enemy hadn't slithered into that furtive silence before the news was broken.

This funeral sure is a long time coming. It's going on and on. You're back at the Institute because you went straight down with a fever on Monday so you're now on antibiotics. Out of danger. Or that danger, at least. Your neutrophil count just keeps going down; soon you'll have no defenses left. If it doesn't come back up in time for the next course of chemo we'll lose you. And in the middle of all this we still have to go to the morgue. The Curie in the morning, Gustave Roussy in the afternoon. I kiss your grandfather's forehead. He's cold and peaceful. I stand silently by his side for a long time with my hand on his, talking to him inside my head. On Thursday he'll be put into his coffin and buried.

Until then your father and I are killing time, and we've found an occupation: we're looking for a babysitter. We loathe the previous one—it's a good diversion. The girl who's been with us for six months didn't show up at Anna's and Nils's schools last Thursday. She didn't call, gave no warning, she simply didn't show up. I was at the Institute, your father was at work, and your brother and sister were forgotten on the sidewalk. Given our situation, she was indispensable to us: she managed the little ones' routine every evening—the school pickup, bath time, homework, and supper—until your father came to take over from me at the Institute. Our messages to her went unanswered for two days. The last of them was sent at eight o'clock on Saturday morning: "Sandrine, we haven't heard from you since Thursday. We're worried. Something really serious must have happened to you for you to leave the kids like this with no warning. Maybe you had an accident? That's all I can think. If you have, tell us if we can help you. If not, you should know that, on top of everything else, the children just lost their grandfather. We don't think it's right to inflict any more upheavals on them. They need security and stability." She called back the same day, clutching at the alibi of an accident that we ourselves had supplied. I don't honestly know whether our intention had been ill-judged or ironic. A bit of both, I think. We'd have liked it to be true but we'd already picked up the scent of something else and it was fun tracking it down.

So she'd been hit by a car, she claimed, when she was on her way to pick the children up on Thursday. She'd been in a coma for two days and had just come out of it. She was feeling much better now and would be back with us on Monday. "In a coma." It's amazing how certain words used in a particular context can take on an unexpected weight. Instead of fading like an echo they seem to keep growing louder once the sentence has been uttered. They become a haunting presence, like a scab standing out on the smooth surface of memory. In the end they're the only thing anyone can see, like an ugly wart in the hollow of a cheek or on the tip of a nose. Coma. Sandrine definitely said coma. I suspected she was lying. In any other circumstances, I'd have savored the implausibility of her miraculous recovery and even joked about it, but in our present situation the lie wouldn't wash. It was obscene. How dare she? A coma. Another one! Why not cancer, leukemia, lymphoma while she was at it?

I was actually very annoyed with myself: I should have anticipated this, I knew, right from the start. From the moment she came to see us last June, sitting on the end of the sofa with her elbows on her knees, a ready answer to every question and her résumé in hand. Too smooth, too perfect, too well prepared for a babysitting job. That too-muchness must have been there for a reason: compensating for a major drawback, a hidden vice, a fundamental shortcoming. Something wasn't right, anyway. A sort of disconnect. I don't know whether it was the gaps in her résumé or those in her teeth that put me on to her. There was a whiff of penury, prison, or street living about it, I told your father at the time. Still, we took her on. In the absence of an objective reason not to, I quashed my doubts. On her first day of work she admitted she lived in a homeless hostel, having spent two months on the streets. A violent, manipulative new stepfather had thrown her out. I decided to help her climb back up the slippery slope by giving her this job and helping her find accommodation. Someone needed to give her a leg up, after all. The early months went well but I was still on my guard, anxious about the harmful effects that her own possible emotional neglect might have on her relationship with my children. I often worked at home anyway, and when I needed to stay at the University of Grenoble overnight your father came home from work a little earlier. But there were no grounds for concern: Sandrine took good care of you and she was kind, patient, and affectionate. We trusted her. Until you got cancer.

She was there the day we received the news. I was too preoccupied to think about it but her lack of empathy shocked me. At first I put it down to surprise and shock, but the next few weeks confirmed my initial reaction: she didn't seem to understand the scale of the ordeal we were facing and deliberately ignored everything you were going through. Sometimes when I was looking after you she would have this strange smile on her face, almost a grimace. One time she came to work sick with the flu; she had a fever. You were at home for a few days in aplasia. I explained that germs were dangerous for you and she should go home, look after herself, and come back when she was better. She didn't understand and didn't want to leave, feeling excluded, rejected. I explained again, at length, but she didn't want to hear it. Her abandonment issues were overriding the facts. I couldn't do this to her, I was discarding her, thinking of no one but my son. She was absolutely right about that. Then for no apparent reason she suddenly changed her tune: now she was the one afraid of abandoning me, she must stay for my sake. Once again I explained that you were at home so I could look after the three of you on my own so long as you weren't in the hospital. In the end she left, got some rest, and came back to work two days later. But something had changed. She seemed less stable, talked about trouble at the hostel, problems with money and relationships. Mostly I noticed that she now smiled openly every time you were mentioned. Two weeks later she vanished.

So I was annoyed with myself when I called her that Saturday. Annoyed because I'd been so credulous, I hadn't listened to my instincts, I'd put you in danger, if not physically, at least psychologically, in the name of some pointless solidarity. I still had room for hope, just a little. Until the lie. Until the coma. On the phone to her, I acted normal, wished her a speedy recovery and arranged to see her the following Monday. That same evening your father and I called every emergency room in Paris to ask whether they'd tended to an unconscious young woman on Thursday. Of course not one of them had. My hope morphed into disappointment and the disappointment into anger. Anger is a stimulating feeling—it gives you an appetite for things, gives you ideas, and a pinch of perversity too. I wanted to see her tie herself in knots with the story she'd spun. Trip herself up, fall flat on her face, and be slowly dragged down into it. Coma. It was never going to take. We called her back, asked a few questions about her accident, and she answered them calmly and clearly. She chose her words carefully and was credible even to connoisseurs. She was good at this, intelligent, and practiced too, most likely. But we were driven on by a heartbreak that intensified our resentment, so we kept going. "Which hospital are you in?" A hesitation, only momentary. She really was talented. "Tenon Hospital." That was enough; the time had come to go into action. "That's convenient, the morgue's quite close. We could come and see you tomorrow when we're done there. Would you prefer flowers or chocolates?" Improbable. I was clearly a less expert liar than she was. Never mind. It was all the more delectable if she grasped the enormity of the suggestion. The aporia of the robbed robber who can't complain. She hesitated longer this time, then said that the doctors had actually said she could go home earlier, on Sunday morning. I offered to pick her up—one last little delight for the road. Because the truth was, I'd had enough of playing games. I had better things to do. Before she'd even concocted a new confabulation, I told her I wasn't fooled. She hung up straightaway and hasn't given a sign of life since. I called her hostel and they didn't know anything about an accident or a coma, but they could tell us that Sandrine hadn't been living there for the last two weeks. She'd moved out.

We activated our network of friends and acquaintances yesterday and we have a lead for a new babysitter. A boy. He

seems a nice, honest, balanced sort. And he starts tomorrow.
So everything's fine. Still, this funeral is a long time coming.

*It rains the day of Jacky's funeral. That's not the worst of
it: that morning Solal has a fever of 103 even though it had
dropped to 100 after two days back in the hospital. That was a
stroke of luck. At the child's request, his parents had negotiated
a half-day leave pass so that he could go to his grandfather's
funeral—he particularly wanted to. The doctors had agreed
to it, despite the fact he was still in total aplasia, on condition
that his temperature had dropped and he wore a mask. As it
is, they can no longer let him out. Solal doesn't understand, he
doesn't want to understand. He cries and screams and yells,
claiming this is the cruelest example of cancer forcing him to
miss out on something. The frustration is unendurable but
there's no choice. His parents listen to his pain, console him,
hug him, and make promises: his maternal grandparents will
come over to be with him this afternoon, friends will film the
ceremony for him, and a stone will be laid on the grave in his
name. He'll be with them in their thoughts and therefore by
proxy. Lise spends the morning at the Institute with her son
while Olivier goes to the morgue at Gustave Roussy to see his
father laid out in his coffin. Later the two of them go home to
Anna and Nils and the four of them—just the four of them—
set off for the cemetery in Bagnolet. It's on the other side of the*

city, the far side of the beltway. It was difficult finding a place to take Jacky's tomb; Paris is overflowing—there's an accommodation crisis from birth right through to death. People have to fight for a place in creches, schools, universities, jobs, apartments, social housing, centers for the disabled, prisons, public transport, leisure centers, hospitals, emergency rooms, obstetrics, pediatrics, geriatrics, oncology, even at the Institute, right down to the cemetery. A shortage of beds, rooms, vaults. A lack of space and funds. And so this funeral is just a little longer in coming as they make their way across Paris.

They finally get there, the last to arrive. Beside the coffin Lise and Olivier each make their own short speech prepared the day before. Olivier speaks first: "Dearest Dad, it's your own special father's day today," and, frequently repeating these words to give him strength, he describes his father's life affectionately, humorously, and poetically. Next Lise talks about Jacky's two lives: the resurrected life after the accident like a supplementary existence and the other life, before, which was glorious, luminous. His youth in Tunisia, his love for Thérèse, their family home, their happy children, the condiments factory where he worked, their friends and travels. It smells of jasmine and olives, spices and laughter. The two speeches end in the same way, with the last words Jacky said to Solal.

It's stopped raining. The children play in the mud between the graves. The coffin is lowered into the ground. Olivier, Lise, Anna, and Nils lay five small white pebbles on the freshly turned earth.

LP

top it! Mom, I want to die. They're hurting me too much. I can't take any more."

You're sitting on the examination table, stripped to the waist, legs dangling, trunk hunched over with a rounded back and your arms crossed on your thighs. The spinous processes of your vertebrae protrude as if about to break through the skin, like spikes along the spine of some fantastical creature. I'm crouching at your feet with my hands on either side of your elbows, desperately trying to communicate some strength to you with this contact that I hope makes you feel safe and secure. For a good ten minutes now we've maintained unbroken eye contact, and your eyes—like your voice—are full of distress.

It's the day of your ordeal, the lumbar puncture, when cerebrospinal fluid is taken using a needle inserted between two vertebrae. It's an essential procedure: it allows the medical team to check that your central nervous system hasn't been affected by the lymphoma. Only experienced doctors can perform it and it requires extreme precision and scrupulous sterilization. You have to submit to this twice a week during each course of chemotherapy. You dread it more than anything else. It has to be said it's quite a process: first there's the whole preparatory protocol that's so solemn that it seems to sanctify the time and the place. The only people in the room are the doctor, the two nurses assisting him, you, and I. We're all wearing protective uniforms of tunics, masks, caps, molded overshoes, and latex gloves. The doctor comes over to where sterilized medical instruments have been laid out religiously in order on a tray, and he goes through a sequence of what look like carefully ordained gestures, like a priest preparing the eucharist. He asks you to keep quiet and perfectly still while the nurses spread nauseous-smelling iodide and saline disinfectant over your skin. Now you're ready for the sacrifice. Next comes the fine hollow needle, about four inches long. Every precaution has been taken so you don't see it but no one can stop you feeling it as it pierces the middle of your back at ninety degrees to your skin. It crosses the dura mater that resists for a moment before letting it penetrate further. When the needle reaches the fluid in the arachnoid cavity the doctor checks that it's securely implanted by slightly withdrawing the detachable stylet that was obstructing the flow. If the positioning is good, droplets form at the end of the needle and the stylet is then completely released, allowing the fluid to flow freely. It's a clear, transparent, colorless liquid that the doctors nickname spring water, a rather beautiful metaphor. At least there's that. It's collected in a number of tubes that are sent straight to the lab.

I don't know how painful the procedure is; opinions vary. At the Institute they tell us it shouldn't hurt. A few minutes beforehand you're given a sedative and they put a patch covered in anesthetizing cream on the area where the puncture is to be made. But we've heard that in the pediatric oncology departments of other hospitals, implantable chambers rather like the port-a-cath are inserted between the vertebrae of young patients so that the needle doesn't have to be reinserted so deeply every time. I can only deduce that it's not a trifling matter. Either way, you're particularly terrified of it. And it hurts you. As for me, I'll readily admit to the physical and psychological trauma of this sharp instrument piercing into you, and the fact that it's going on behind your back certainly adds to your feeling of impotence. This helplessness aggravates your distress, which increases your fear, which heightens your pain. So far, though, we've managed to get through it. This is the seventh lumbar puncture you've had and, with experience, we've perfected a preparation routine that means you now hardly feel a thing. To achieve this I've borrowed and adapted the hypnosis technique I used for your first surgical intervention, and this consists in replacing the anesthetizing patch—which is too superficial to cope with this invasive procedure—with a mental one that we picture as very thick. Where the one acts on the surface, the other operates deep down. This imaginary object is constructed by verbal suggestion, using basic rhetorical tools, repetitions, and accumulations. But it does need to achieve such a density in your mind that it virtually comes into being, and that's why it needs to come from your inner world alone. I just try to help you develop the image of it by asking a series of questions. I know you can do this, and that's partly because of your age: childhood offers a sort of natural proximity between the real world and fantasy worlds, allowing for free exchanges between them. Besides, you happen to be remarkably sensitive, creative, and attuned to language, all qualities that have made you particularly receptive to this technique once I explained it to you and you accepted the principle.

The truth is, I have to admit I know nothing about hypnosis; I don't even realize that ideodynamic techniques have been used for pain relief since the nineteenth century. I haven't learned any, practiced any, or even experienced any myself. So, beyond the trust I have in your intelligence, it takes a degree of nerve on my part to suggest such a fanciful solution to your suffering. My interest in literature is no stranger to the concepts: I've been working on fictional, imaginary worlds for twenty years now and, therefore, know about the power of words and visualization. And the element of truth in them. It could be said that I believe in them. The purpose of today's visit, however, isn't to create something but to protect. And soothe. I just want to take you someplace where you won't be in pain.

"Solal, I'm going to put an anesthetizing patch on you. What shape would you like it to be?"

"Square."

"Solal, I'm going to put a square anesthetizing patch on you. What size should it be?"

"Four inches each side."

"Solal, I'm going to put a four-inch-square anesthetizing patch on you. What color are you picturing it?"

"Black, it's black."

The shape and size don't change much from one lumbar puncture to another, but the color varies to match your morale.

"Solal, I'm going to put a black four-inch-square anesthetizing patch on you. What should it be made of?"

The choice of material is vital. Sometimes you prefer it soft, smooth, and comforting—cotton wool, feather, fur, silk—and sometimes rough, angular, and hostile—stone, metal, leather, horn—depending on whether you view the patch as a sedating balm laid over a deep wound or as a protective shield against an external aggressor.

"It's made of steel, with very pointy spikes on it in lots of different sizes. Some of them have gold on the tips, some of them ice, and some fire." You seem to be in defensive mode today.

"Solal, I'm going to put a black four-inch-square anesthetizing patch made of steel onto you with very pointy spikes in lots of different sizes, with gold, ice, and fire on the tips. Can I put it onto you now?"

"Yes. Go ahead."

I carefully pick up the invisible object, mindful that I mustn't damage it with a wrong move or one word too many. It's fragile because it's virtual. The slightest thing could damage it. I bring it up to the small of your back and you give a little shiver at the feel of it. You've imagined it so hard that you can feel it and it now exists. I put the lower edge of it under your second lumbar vertebra, trying to place it perfectly symmetrically over your spine. First I apply the left-hand corner, holding it firmly in place with one of my thumbs while the other slides slowly to the right, turns through a ninety-degree angle, and goes up the side to the top of the square. Now it's attached on two sides. Then with the back of my free hand I smooth the rest of it down in a diagonal action toward the top left-hand corner so that it's completely stuck to your skin. I describe each move I make and my words stand in for your eyes. I ask whether it feels right and you say it does. The lumbar puncture can begin. You're ready.

It worked every other time and the child coped with the ordeal. The patch was literally incarnated in its anesthetic role, it became so tangible that the child would frequently ask his mother to take it off once the procedure was over so that it wouldn't be uncomfortable. In fact, it's working well on this occasion too. At least at first. This LP is even looking likely to go well: this time it's a qualified female pediatrician in charge of the procedure and not, as is often the case, an intern. She introduces the needle coolly, it plies in, and the child stays motionless. All at once the mother has a strange feeling, not that something worrying will happen—a scream, sudden accelerated movements, rushed instructions, some sign of an emergency—but precisely because nothing's happening. The pediatrician doesn't turn back to the tray to set down the stylet, nor does she ask to be handed a tube to collect the cerebrospinal fluid. Nothing. She does nothing. She just stays there peering at the child's back. Perfectly still, perfectly silent. Only her lips seem to move, emitting a long, slow exhalation through the mask. At the same time she lowers her eyelids. This goes on for some while. Lise couldn't say how long. It's just too long. Then the pediatrician opens her eyes and turns them almost imperceptibly to the nurses. She seems a little pale, mutters a few inaudible phrases. Judging by the team's reaction, the news isn't great. Next, she leans toward the child to speak to him directly, while the older of the two nurses gently strokes his head. "I'm so sorry, Solal," she says. "I need to take out this needle and insert it again. It hasn't worked." Lise doesn't immediately grasp what this means, she doesn't anticipate the problem. She's never considered how long her virtual patch remains effective. She's never wondered, for example, what would happen if it had to be used twice in a row without recourse to a new hypnosis session in between. To be frank, it hasn't occurred to her that an imaginary object *might be single-use, expending all its energy like a battery. But here they are coping with the unexpected, with a problem. Not a chink or a fissure or even a hairline crack in the system but still enough to bring it tumbling down.*

Lise doesn't think and doesn't anticipate what's coming. She keeps her eyes focused on her son. First she just notices that tears are forming along the child's eyelids, then she hears a little whimpering sound, a sort of high-pitched keening, when the second needle pierces his skin. Time stands still once more. Everything freezes again. The pediatrician hunched over the child. The nurses stroking his head. Mother and son looking into each other's eyes. Entirely focused on her child, the mother doesn't suspect the doctor's shaking hands, her hesitant gestures, or her repeated failure to insert the needle. The sweat trickling down her temples. But she can make out the progressive increase in pain, visible in the scars that the doctor's efforts are tracing over her child's face. His features contorting, the furrows forming as their topography alters. Something's wrong. Is this a human failing (lack of practice, a wave of tiredness, a rush of emotion), some specific element (the child being particularly tense or in the wrong position, a faulty instrument), or any inextricable combination of multiple factors? What does the cause matter—the dura mater is resisting, the needle won't go in, and the pediatrician's repeated attempts to get it through are hurting the child. The patch has stopped working. Maybe it's stopped even existing. Solal tolerates the agony in silence until he eventually screams.

"Stop it! Mom, I want to die. They're hurting me too much. I can't take any more."

The child doesn't move; he keeps his back bent, his head lowered, and his eyes wide open, but his entire body tenses and hardens when he screams. His fists on his thighs are clenched, the knuckles going white and his nails digging into his palms. Then he starts moaning quietly, intoning a barely articulated "Mommy" with each new attempt to insert the needle. The time for hypnosis is over. It's failed. There's no room now for imagination. Pain has closed the door to all that. Tenderness and reasoning are all that remain—the one uses hands and eyes to console, caress, and soothe; the other explains, encourages, reassures, and promises that this torture is nearly over. "This has to be done. Don't forget it's to make you better. It'll be over soon. Look right into my eyes. Take my hands and squeeze them. Breathe slowly. There, there, there. That's it. I'm right here." Not for a moment does the mother take her eyes off her son's. Crouching at his feet with her head tipped back and her hands crushed in his, she grafts herself onto him. Does she hope some part of the pain will leave his body and extend into hers to find a new space in which to spread and a new prey to seize? Does she think that by doing this she can offer herself as a substitute for the torment? Taking her son's place, claiming his pain. A pointless, arrogant ambition that fools no one, not even Lise. Because she knows: in the end everyone is alone in their ordeals. How very long those minutes feel with the child's suffering reverberating in his mother's heart.

Meanwhile the pediatrician is still hitting a snag but she doggedly keeps trying. It's unbearable. One of the nurses, the younger one, can't take any more. She sways and the other nurse has to help her out of the room so she doesn't faint in front of the child. Lise can't remember her face or her name but what she can still see is the back of her neck receding through the doorway and on it a tattoo of three little black stars in a vertical line. The last vestiges of imagination escaping. Paradoxically, this desertion by one of their number gives the small group a renewed energy. Each of them individually thinks that he or she isn't the type to give up. So Solal holds out, Lise holds out, and the team holds out. And the time comes when it's over. It feels almost incongruous. Why now rather than earlier? Either way, it's too late. Just as the pediatrician is telling the child that she's withdrawn the needle, the mother suddenly stands up, thanks the team, kisses her son, drops his hand and their eye contact, and leaves the room without another word. She runs aimlessly, hopelessly, pointlessly. She can tell she's going to cry. She wants to get away, find somewhere hidden, out of sight, out of reach, out of it all. She finds refuge in the outpatient department, in the small "parents' room," which is mercifully empty. Never mind the dolphins on the walls, the fake porthole, and the leatherette seats. All that matters is being alone. And the floor too. It's somewhere to lie down. On her stomach at first, facedown as if trying to melt into the floor, be swallowed up by it. Disappear. For a long time. Silent and motionless. Inert. Then she lets the sobs fill *and swell and detonate at will, blasting into the air. Bellowing her pain with her nose crushed and her mouth twisted against the floor. Thumping it with her fists. Then feeling the substance of it resisting her, marveling at how solid and smooth it is, experiencing each point of contact. Finding some comfort in it. And eventually curling up on the warm linoleum, her back rounded, her legs bent, and her head between her hands. Breathing slowly. Listening to the to and fro of her breathing. Waiting, just a little longer.*

After that there are no more failed lumbar punctures; they go without a hitch. Everything is back to normal. I prepare you using hypnosis, the imaginary patch works again, the intern proceeds with precision, the first needle is all it takes, and you're not in too much pain. On the other hand, I've stopped going into the room with you for LPs. Too shocking for a mother, I've been told. And you now refuse to let anyone touch your back. For years you won't be able to bear being stroked or massaged there. At least you no longer want to die. There is that.

BORA-BORA

Listen to me. One day it'll all be over, Solal. Don't look at the needle. You'll be free. You'll be cured. Don't take any notice of the nurses. Then all five of us will go on a trip. To Bora-Bora. Breathe slowly. It's a gorgeous, sun-filled island on the other side of the world, in Polynesia. Close your eyes. Imagine an extinct volcano surrounded by a turquoise lagoon and protected from the high seas by a barrier of coral. Let yourself go. There's only a narrow passage through the circle of reef. You get through it in a dugout canoe. Give me your hand. From the boat you can see through the transparent water to the incredible depths below, the white sand, the rocks and the multicolored fish. You can dive in. Come on, come with me. What's that salty smell? It's the sea. That prickling against your chest? The spines of a sea urchin. The line rolling down your body? Some seaweed perhaps, or a stray tendril from a jellyfish. There's a sea turtle over there. Can you see? We're lucky, they're rare. Follow it for a while. Careful. They have weak hearts. You mustn't frighten them. Do you know that this island's real name is Pora-Pora, the "firstborn"? It was made just for you. The Tahitians also call it *mai te pora*, "created by the gods." Everything's fine, my darling. The puncture's over. We'll all go to Bora-Bora.

MORPHEUS

I t's nighttime. You can't get to sleep. It hovers close to you in many guises, skimming you with its silent wing, gliding over you with its opiate caresses. But never succeeding in carrying you away. There's too much pain and this resists the darkness, boredom, and exhaustion. Even the morphine. Your thumb keeps pressing the switch on the pump, which now refuses to give you another dose. You've had a succession of boluses to no avail; you've gone over the pain relief threshold many times. It's a terrible disappointment. You've reached level III, the strongest analgesics, and were promised you would have control. You thought it would be total control, pain relief connected directly to your central catheter, the height of autonomy. Your body in closed circuit with the poison and its antidote in the same pipework: PCA in the PAC— patient-controlled analgesic in the port-a-cath. With your finger on the button, triggering soothing injections as and when you need them. It's stopped working and you keep jabbing at the button. You wail and cry and roar in anger and despair. You howl at the injustice of it. It certainly is an unequal battle: safety introduces limits, whereas the pain can deploy its forces at will.

A nurse comes into the room and reprimands you. "It's not a joystick, Solal, stop." She's not wrong there, if you think about it, there's no joy in any of this. But there's one way in which she is wrong, on a fact that you acknowledged a long time back, and it's precisely because of this fact, because a part of you no longer has any place in childhood games, that you've been trusted to administer your pain relief yourself. You're no more addicted to the gadget than you are to the drugs it releases: you're just in terrible pain and can't think how to deal with it.

Game over. Your pump is unplugged. You failed on the brink of autonomy and must go back to the previous level. From now on you'll be given morphine on an ad hoc basis and on the oncologist's decision. A long process strewn with pitfalls: calling the nurse, your request being registered, your prescription checked, the injection prepared, then administered, and the drug being absorbed. Nearly an hour between you expressing pain and the treatment becoming effective. And it isn't enough, anyway.

It's therapeutic aporia. Sleeping pills and tranquilizers take over from analgesics and knock you out. There's no other remedy offered for your pain, and your body is left like that: sedated, alone, abandoned, ravaged by torments way beyond its scope. Your time trickles by like this, in a semiconscious state in which you try to find an illusory deliverance. You tiptoe softly away from yourself and eventually fall asleep, at last. A heavy, deep, dreamless sleep. You wake much later, disoriented. The searing pain is still faithfully there. It's just changed and has colonized your brain, whispering something in your ear. You can't make it out at all, don't even recognize this pain. You can't say where it hurts; in fact, you no longer even know that anything does hurt. And that's when you're invited into the secrets room. Someone's waiting for you there, at the far end of the corridor, waiting to get you to talk and to listen to you. The hope is that this will help you reclaim your own body with language, transforming pain into words, suffering into sentences. Describing the nausea, vomiting, mucositis, myalgia, weakness, and tiredness. Saying "I'm in pain," "I can't go on," "I can't take any more." Saying "I." Sketching out in your mind the contours of your vanished self. But you can't do it. You sit there mutely, as if detached from yourself. Dissociated.

Your body on one side, your psyche on the other. Morphine here, psychotherapy there. A strange duality. There seems to be a missing link in the chain, a missing intermediary. Before asking how you feel about all this, no one taught you to listen to what was going on in your body. They're trying to make you speak a language you don't know. But there are plenty of ways you could be taught it, plenty of things you could be shown that would help you converse with your sick body. Laying you down in a calm place away from prying eyes, inviting you to turn your attention to yourself and notice your sensations, explore the places where the pain concentrates and those it spares, feel all the parts of you around it that breathe, feed, function, and still live perfectly. What does the technique matter—sophrology, hypnosis, meditation, or relaxation. Every decade has its fads. They may occasionally be raised to the level of dogma or debased into charlatanism but that doesn't invalidate them. Used as therapeutic supports, they could help you, if not to increase your resistance, at least to gather it together; and to feel that the affected areas haven't dismantled all of you. They could help you rediscover a reassuring coherence behind the distortions of the disease. Maybe then you'd succeed in talking about it in the secrets room.

I'm not qualified, it's not my job. I'm bound to be making lots of mistakes but I give it a try. A mother's caresses aren't enough in the face of so much pain. You need to be brought gently back to your own inner resources. Day after day I try to be the mirror in which you can see the continuation of who you are. I reflect the breadth of your imagination, the power of your creativity, the virtues of your humor, and the liveness of your articulacy. I transmit to you the little that I know. Self-hypnosis, self-massage, self-relaxation. The important thing is to give you back the autonomy stolen by cancer. In order to achieve this, I need to be available without interfering, ready to intervene if I'm needed, but also prepared to be forgotten. I need to be there but not too much, like an invisible sentinel, a benevolent ghost. When you wish that you could play with your friends, laugh, bicycle, and go to school like you used to. When you refuse to eat, when you're in pain, when you scream, when you shout, and when you groan. When you want to give up altogether. It's a delicate balance to strike. I sometimes struggle but I stay on course. It's the only option. On your last day in the hospital one of the psychologists confirms this fact in the privacy of her office: "Well done," she says. "Well done to you and your son. Our whole team is full of admiration. You managed to be with him the whole time but you still allowed him his freedom and independence. And he knew how to make the most of that." I'll take the compliment for what it's worth. We didn't have any choice, anyway. We absolutely had to put you back in touch with your dreams.

YOU SHALL BE A MAN,
MY SON

They're at home. The child is resting in his bedroom, the room in which he's spent so little time since his tenth birthday. The landline rings and the Institute's number comes up on the screen. It's the only number that still uses this line, anyway. The mother's body tenses, suggesting that this isn't good news. Her body must be forgiven, its memory has been corrupted, it can't be helped. Lise shudders, she's frightened; her son had another PET scan this morning. Yet another. They have a meeting with the oncologist the next day to discuss the results. Why then this premature phone call? Lise waits. Three, four rings. Pointless. It doesn't stop. She picks up. And it's him, Dr. O. She's surprised, he's never called them himself. Her heart's beating so fast it might stop, particularly as the doctor doesn't sound like his usual self. His voice is loaded with emotion, his words seem to wobble.

What's he saying? She doesn't immediately understand. Not that the doctor's words aren't clear, but she's not really there. She can't help thinking back to when it all began, to the beginnings of this evil, to the very first phone call from Dr. G. That was months ago. An eternity. She was in the same room, *in the same place, with the same phone in her hand. But in another life. "Can you hear me, Mrs. M?" The doctor's aware of her absence. "Yes, yes, I'm listening," she rallies. "Don't worry, I'm calling with good news. It's not every day... So I couldn't resist the pleasure of calling you. I couldn't wait till tomorrow to tell you. The PET scan is perfect. The chemotherapy has worked. We can consider your son to be in remission already. We weren't expecting a result like this for weeks. It's unhoped-for." The mother could swear the oncologist's voice cracked on those last words. Yes, he's definitely lost some of his usual distance. Proof, if any were needed, that it is only there for his protection. Meanwhile, Lise's head is spinning. She's still not sure she's understood. She knows perfectly well this isn't about a total recovery. It's far too soon. It's more as if the cancer has been lulled to sleep but could wake at any moment. But surely that's a first victory? She feels its significance without gauging its scope. She thinks she might well be sobbing. Even narrowly opening the door to hope like this has weakened her defenses. She in turn is lowering her guard. She and Dr. O have never been so close. If he were here, she'd hug him. Galvanized by the news, she asks for more. For too much, already. "Can he come home, then? I mean for good?" "No, we still need to follow the protocol through to the end, to be absolutely sure. He'll come back in two months, as planned. But this is very encouraging." His voice is reverting to its usual tone: Neutral. Medical. It brings the conversation back in line. Restrains it and confines it. And now Lise understands the*

vital role this neutrality plays. She won't be asking any more
questions. Never mind. She too puts her armor back on. Ready
simply to savor the good news.

I think I just said your name out loud. With the joy, the
relief, the triumph of it. I think you came running. You
always hear everything so you know, you know the phone
rang, you know it was the Institute, perhaps you even know
it was Dr. O. But you don't know what he told me. You try
to read it in my eyes and the way I move. And you guess
before I even tell you. We're both sitting on the edge of my
bed, and I'm holding your hands in mine.

"Oh, Solal...that was your oncologist. The PET
scan was perfect. The lymphoma's gone. Do you understand, it's gone. Nothing left. Do you understand? Do you
understand?"

You throw yourself in my arms, burrowing your head
against my shoulder. I can feel that you're sobbing. I stop
talking, stop moving, hold my breath. I don't want to risk
disturbing what's going on inside you, from you to you, at
this particular moment. I leave you to experience it alone, in
the most secret part of you. Where no one else has access.

How long do we stay here in this silent, motionless embrace? I have no idea. Time doesn't matter anymore. But I
have a strange feeling when you sit back up: it's generated

by your eyes, the way they stare intently at me, and developed by the way you hold yourself, drawing back slightly, straight-backed, head held high with an aloof sort of grace. Then it's confirmed by what you say. Still mingled with tears, your words prove just how fully you understand. All of it. Absolutely all of it. And they imply everything you've been holding back until now. Everything you hid behind childish tears, grievances, joys, and games. Everything you disguised behind the routine gestures of everyday life. Your clear awareness of the danger. Your constant, needling fear of dying. They also talk about the future that you can suddenly allow yourself to envision again, not that you deny the uncertainties. I have nothing to add, nothing to explain to you. We're speaking the same language, communicating as equals. You're ten years old and you're still my little boy but in this moment, in this exchange of laughter, tears, hope, and doubts, I feel as if I'm seeing you differently. Older, more mature, almost adult. With a glance, I appraise who it is that this illness has made of you, and who it will allow you to become. And in this wonderful, fleeting moment I'm quite sure of it: you shall be a man, my son. In a way, you already are.

END?

A few more months and the protocol goes on, subjugating everything to its purpose. It ignores nights, weekends, and holidays. It ignores suffering, exhaustion, rebellion, and abdication. It even ignores its own successes. It goes ahead as planned, unwavering. To the very end. Its formulation is governed by rigorously precise calculations, the product of years of research, theoretical advance, and experimental practices. A combination of medical literature, clinical observation, statistics, and consensus conferences, presiding over the choice of molecules, their dosage, and the duration of their use. The calibrated chemistry of experienced researchers. How many children before their son were treated for longer, more aggressively, and less effectively? How many had to be lost in order to get the treatment right? How many dead children have informed this protocol? And how many more are there to come? How many more will be saved precisely because of these current failures? How many will survive thanks to the aimless wanderings this child has endured? In five, ten, fifteen years, the treatment will be shorter, less invasive, more successful, and perhaps even superfluous. So much evil for so much good. A long chain of therapeutic progress in which every patient is a link, both a part of it and its beneficiary.

Science can pursue its journey; fate always wins. It's fate that decides where, what, and when. A little sooner, it would have been a lost cause. A little later, there would have been no risk. It's better not to think about it and get on with doing what needs to be done.

And so, willingly blind, they all comply with the protocol. It's regulated like the staves on music paper and is the master in charge of time, orchestrating lives. Resistance is futile. Its rhythm atomizes time, subdividing it into successive actions. Six one-week courses of chemotherapy, six consultations with the oncologist, six three-week periods of aplasia, twelve lumbar punctures, thirty-six blood counts, 120 days of nausea, 480 hours of fever. Sometimes a break. Sometimes a recovery. Millions of seconds lost. The present keeps on getting longer for the parents and their child. They don't do the sums, don't think about the countdown. They just keep moving forward along a semblance of a straight line.

And then one day it stops. It happens all of a sudden, and they don't know why. Everything still seems the same: the lack of hair, the pallor, the exhaustion, the low bodyweight. And yet this is the last consultation, the one that allows the child to leave. They can go home; the treatment's over. They almost look surprised.

————

Just like on the first day, we're sitting in the consulting room with you in the middle and us on either side, flanked by two nurses. Like on the first day, Dr. O has rolled around in his chair to face us. Like on the first day, he leans his upper body toward us and crosses his legs, revealing the top of his left sock under the hem of his pants. But it's obvious something has changed and it can't be just that there aren't pictures on the sock. It has to be said that with no coyote or Road Runner it does look very sober, but still. There must be something else. Perhaps a familiarity in the tone of voice and choice of words, an obvious closeness. We are struck afresh by the character and depth of the relationship we've developed with this man without even realizing it. We haven't seen him much but he has worked in the shadows every step of the way to come to this moment. Every procedure on your body, every test to which it's been submitted, every treatment it's been given, every molecule that's penetrated it, was conceived, measured, decided, and instructed by this man. And here we are again, sitting facing him and waiting. Like on the first day. Except that this time we understand what he's saying. We can suddenly see all the months that have gone by as a whole. A period in parentheses is coming to an end.

The treatment is over, there'll be no more green and white pouches, no more port-a-cath, no more pump, no more drip pole, no more tubes, no more calls in the middle of the night. No more lumbar punctures, no more morphine, no more tranquilizers, no more sedatives, no more antiemetics, no more antibiotics. No more aplasia, no more alopecia, no more mucositis, no more vomiting, no more fevers, no more infections, no more pain. We can put away the protective masks, antiseptics, and hygiene precautions. Put away chemotherapy and its whole pharmacopeia. Put away the protocol. Your hair will grow back, you'll start growing again, and your strength will return. You'll even be able to go back to school in a few weeks. This summer you'll go on vacation.

There. It's over.

Over? That would be good. The End. Like at the movies. A clean, clear ending with no tomorrows. Roll the credits. The End...and why not the happy ending of trashy films? The doctor sits the parents and child down opposite him. He stays silent for a moment, his face unreadable, just to stage-manage the moment of surprise. The dramaturgy of suspense is established. The camera simulates dizziness with a circular tracking shot, then finds an anchor point, zooming in on the couple's intertwined hands. The silence is slightly oppressive. The game is to whip up some fear even though everyone knows these stories always end well. Freeze frames of different eye contact: the parents to the doctor, the doctor to the parents, and all three to the child. The tension builds and the silence fills with music. There's a predominance of chords, tremolos from just violins and cellos, a tenuous fabric of sound. Then the score becomes more complex and other instruments join in as the sound builds. The symphony swells and the doctor makes the most of this crescendo to start speaking. He mentions the latest test; he's going to deliver his judgment. The tension is at its peak. A close-up on the tears welling in the mother's eyes, or the father's, or both. Fortissimo. It's heartrending. When the final cadence resolves into a harmonious chord, the results ring out: the child is saved. Good has triumphed over evil. Exhausted by two hours of pathos, the viewer cries. They're crying on-screen too, hugging and congratulating each other. Or, better still, they stay frozen in their seats, dignified and profound, exchanging silent looks laden with meaning. A final tableau celebrates the return to normality: the prodigal son come home to the fold, surrounded by his family, his friends, and his dog, all of them gathered together and deliriously happy. They're playing soccer on a spanking green lawn in front of an immaculate house. The final slow-motion shot ends on the child's face as it breaks into a triumphant smile against the azure sky. Roll the credits. The End.

Actually, it's not really the end. It's "to be continued," as they say. True, there are no traces left of cancer, but that still doesn't mean you're cured. And no one has thought to raise that possibility. For now you're simply in remission. That's a lot but also not a lot. In any event, not enough for us to feel completely free. The word "remission" has barely been spoken before notions such as rest, relaxation, and respite are overshadowed by less pleasing terms: recurrence, readmission. Relapse. We need only listen to Dr. O to understand: "For now," he says, "we just need to monitor." The sentence sounds incomplete. Monitor what exactly? A pointless question. In reality we have no trouble grasping what that absence of an object means. A partial victory, an unfinished war. The villain hasn't had its last word. It may be only sleeping. It could hunker down there in secret and wait for us to lower our guard before attacking again. We need to stay on the alert.

We feel awkward talking about it in front of you so we don't interrupt and let the doctor carry on with what he has to say. He maps out how the months and years to come will proceed with regular appointments, clinical and technical tests, and carefully devised follow-ups. It's no longer treatment, for sure, but it's still part of the protocol. Surveillance has been substituted for chemotherapy with all the same precision and rigor. Yet again our future is reduced to a succession of moments. The final objective isn't mentioned once. The doctor settles instead for explaining the process that can achieve it, putting the unsayable into a series of actions.

You're not fooled. How could you be? You want things to be spoken out loud and, while we sit in silence, you're the one asking questions. "Could it come back?" As usual, Dr. O replies directly: "Yes. The risk is minimal but there is still a risk." This isn't enough for you; we can tell there's something else. You're thinking and we encourage you to talk—now's the time, it's our last consultation, you mustn't come out of here with any doubts...they could potentially be more tragic than the truth. "And what if it comes back?" I think of the very early days and the "It can be treated." I remember Anna and how she lucidly flushed out the uncertainty: "And what if it isn't treated?" We can no longer pretend there aren't any ifs; no one would believe it. "Well," the doctor replies, "then we'd have to go back to the protocol and start chemotherapy again." You show no emotion; you're not shocked or devastated, you don't even seem surprised. You're thinking. "Actually, I have another question." You seem to be searching for the right words or, to be more precise, trying to marshal your thoughts. "So...I was wondering...If the lymphoma comes back, would the chemo work again, like it did this time?" We sure weren't expecting that, the thought hadn't occurred to us. You've projected yourself further than we had. And, truth be told, we don't know the answer. I secretly pray that it's affirmative and, if it isn't, that the doctor will lie to you. Just once, this once. Just now. But lying doesn't seem to be part of the protocol. Without missing a beat, he looks you right in the eye and says, "No, there are absolutely no guarantees it will. Sometimes it doesn't work anymore." Like on the first day, I take the blow right in the stomach. Like on the first day, I sag visibly, and so does your father. You meanwhile sit impassively.

The doctor takes a sheet of paper and draws two concentric circles in pencil. "This, Solal, is a cancerous cell. It's surrounded by a membrane and it's this protective layer that the chemotherapy breaks through to destroy the cell." The tip of the pencil mimes the process, zigzagging around the outer circle, and jabbing at it repeatedly. It's dumb but it reminds me of an old toothpaste ad back in the eighties. A simple stylized image of a tooth, the base dotted with little marks: "It's here, between the tooth and the gum, that bacteria attack." I smile incongruously. Unlike the fictional characters in the commercial, medical teams don't have magic erasers to rub out harmful cells. Instead, Dr. O keeps going with his pencil, repeatedly circling the membrane. Once, twice, ten times around the outside. There's something compulsive and distressing about it. The line is growing thicker. Soon the only thing we can see is this circle with its swollen circumference. "Sometimes," the doctor says, "the outer layer is different and impossible to penetrate. In these cases chemotherapy doesn't work." A pause. Then he sits up and adds, "but that's rare."

There. We started with one diagram and we're finishing with another. At the start, an arrow heading toward an uncertain future. The chronological line of your torture, a half line reaching into infinity. Now we have a circle with impenetrable boundaries closing in on further uncertainties. The tiny, absurd, ridiculous, but still insistent eventuality of an incurable relapse. We've come full circle. There's nothing left to say.

Still, Dr. O asks whether there's anything else you'd like to know. You sit in silence. It seems you've heard enough. Then, as with previous consultations, he asks you to go back to the waiting room alone because, he says, he wants to talk to us about boring stuff you won't find interesting. He seems to have more of a gift for euphemism than lying. After you've left, he sits back down facing us and sighs.

"That's not a child's question," he says.

"Excuse me?" We don't immediately understand.

"What Solal asked at the end. It's not a child's question."

"What do you mean?"

"His question about chemotherapy. He can't have come up with that on his own. Someone must have given him the idea."

I'm dumbstruck. I despise that "someone," the pronoun of passive denunciation, veiled reproach, unspoken truths, and hidden meanings. The indefinite neutrality of cowards. Besides, his assumption is wrong and displays a blatant misapprehension. I'm amazed that such an experienced doctor should make this mistake. The pediatrician in him must have forgotten what the oncologist can't ignore: these children are no longer really children. They have an adult disease, an old person's disease even, and it makes them precocious. And the medical team are to some extent instrumental in this forced acceleration of their maturing process. They may not be directly responsible for it but they at least make the most of it, often contribute to it, and sometimes, truth be told, rely on it. The insistence on giving these children the truth, information, and autonomy is commendable in itself but, pushed to the extreme, it inflicts yet more constraints on them. Their caregivers so want to treat them as individuals in their own right that they forget they are in fact dealing with children. They tell them everything, or nearly. They tell them too much. And the very things the children are not told are what they know most clearly and dread the most. They're taught to name, understand, and question their pathologies. They're given pamphlets, DVDs, and comics explaining the causes, the mechanisms, and the treatments. They're given endless contradictory instructions, inviting them to look after themselves while they're being subjected to treatments, to stand on their own two feet while submitting to whatever's inflicted on them, to be both active players and patients. The fact that the teaching tools bear the codes of childhood and that everyone tries to find the right words to explain things doesn't change anything. These children know. And knowing removes them from childhood.

That's how a sick kid gets through the day, with a cuddly toy in one hand and a drip pole in the other, shouldering responsibility not only for some of the caregiving incumbent on adults, but also for some share of their anxieties. He knows. He knows the names of the treatments, the molecules, and the medical equipment; knows their desired outcome, their form and function; recognizes their needs and anticipates their side effects. All on his own, he will remember to gargle with mouthwash several times a day to avoid mucositis. He alone will identify a rise in temperature long before the official thermometer check is scheduled. He alone will notice that the rate of a drip has slowed or a dose of painkillers been forgotten. He knows. He understands the complex organization of the department, is familiar with the timetable of staff shifts, anticipates when the nurses won't be available, intuits the staff's priorities, compensates for their heavy workloads and their possible moments of weakness. He alone will fetch a clean kidney bowl, a glass of water, or a drug that's taking too long to arrive. He alone will stop the shrill alarm signaling a malfunction in his drip or low battery power in the pump. And still alone he might deliberately set off the same alarm in the middle of the night to wake a parent sharing his bedroom and whose snoring is stopping him sleeping, or to bring an emergency to the attention of a caregiver oblivious to his calls. He alone will go help a young neighbor who can't get up to reach a bib, a teddy bear, a hanky, or a spit bowl. In fact in any eventuality he alone will decide to avoid disturbing the already overworked staff unless it's an absolute necessity. He knows. He knows the limits of pain relief, and the limits of therapy too. He knows that medicine isn't an exact science, and that it doesn't always win. He knows he might die. Alone, he will think about this, or make every effort not to think about it. Alone, he will decide to stay quiet and keep his upsetting questions to himself. Alone, he will pretend he knows nothing.

No one suggested that question to you, for sure. Your words are neither a child's nor an adult's. They're ageless. They don't belong to normal life. They're the words of a sick person, the words of a cancer patient. And the oncologist replied coolly, technically, as he would to a cancer patient. You know. Like the others. You know. Mostly what you know is that no one ever knows. And you sometimes allow yourself to say so.

As on previous occasions, at least the child is spared the rest of the conversation. This is the parents' time. When they are left alone with the doctor and can ask their questions. When— unwitting or valorous—they can peer a little further over the abyss and gauge its depth. It's the moment of harsh truths. They understand. This departure isn't really a departure at all. It certainly is easier to come into the Institute than to leave it. So they'll be back; often and for months to come. Then a little less frequently for years. And then even less frequently for years after that. For a long time, a very long time. Long enough for their son to end up returning without them. This childhood illness will follow him into adulthood, might even keep following him when they are no longer of this world. Exactly how long will it go on? That's not clear; the oncologist hesitates, wavering between two possibilities, tracing out very divergent paths for the future.

On the one hand, they will soon need to check the effects of the chemotherapy on his fertility. In this instance, the monitoring will stop when his first baby is conceived, or when such an eventuality proves impossible. So the question of infertility remains unanswered, like a debt taken out on the future, leaving the former patient potentially overdrawn as a result of his recovery. Lymphoma is insatiable, a perverse ogre not satisfied with gobbling up his childhood, and who years later wants to attack his progeny. It may be shocking but it's not insurmountable. There's room for hope. In this particular area the debts are quite often written off. Time passes and wounds heal. Nature reclaims its rights. Kronos goes ahead and regurgitates his offspring. If this doesn't happen, all is not lost: medicine and society have made advances to right this wrong. There can be assisted reproductive technology, donors, tubes, gametes, and inseminations. There can be adoption, files, authorizations, and international flights. There may be failed efforts, disappointed expectations, tensions in the relationship, specialists, and advisers, and highs and lows. There may be failures. What does it matter: there will be a future and aspirations for another future beyond that. One way or another *this child who risked no longer being here at all will live a full and whole life. Teenager, adult, senior, old man. For his parents, nothing matters but this assurance, this vanishing point of remission opening onto the horizon of full recovery.*

Still there is no guarantee that this goal will ever be reached. Beneath their rigorous exterior, the oncologist's words sometimes become less clear. As he charts out the years to come, a quite different cartography is also implicit, allowing room for the fear that they may return to the starting point. In this respect, then, the monitoring protocol seems to have no end. It's "for life," the doctor confirms. A terrifyingly figurative expression that makes the parents shudder. Does that mean that the danger itself also goes on forever? The question certainly needs asking. And in turn triggers another scientific explanation, as technical and clearly constructed as the last, although its radical opposite. It reveals the fact that even a long time after recovery there's still potential for secondary cancers. Having been affected at such a young age and for unexplained reasons, the child is classified as being "at risk." Cold statistics seize power again and the statement is painful: here they are on their way out, and just as they are about to be released, right on the doorstep, they still have to suffer this blow. And it's followed by another even crueler one dealt in a dispassionate voice by a double-edged weapon. A merciless weapon in the form of a biochemical explanation. This child will need monitoring "for life" because some of the molecules he received during his treatment are mutagens, so the very thing that saved him could, in the future, destroy him. Of course, the oncologist reminds them, the risk-benefit ratio is in their favor. Of course, these cases of secondary cancers are very rare. Everything is relative. But fate can dress itself up in reassuring statistics as much as it likes—it's too late. Something that should have been left unsaid has been formulated. And nothing can now silence it again. The image of their son bald once more, pierced by needles, draped in tubes, repeating his childhood battle as an adult, will now always superimpose itself over the image of a vigorous, flourishing young man with dreams of fatherhood. The parents have also been told too much.

We did it, we got here. We're on the threshold, ready to go, to leave the Institute and go back into the outside world. The doctor stands facing us, shaking us warmly by the hand.

"And now," he says, "forget about us. See you in three weeks for your next appointment."

The message is as clear as it's contradictory and there are elements of a challenge and of the absurd in this paradox. It single-handedly encapsulates the complex makeup of the months to come: we survived and now we need to start living again.

Maybe the doctor's right. Maybe for now that just means forgetting and waiting. Forgetting while we wait, forgetting that we're waiting, month after month, for the fear to come back. And, in the breaks between, making the most of newfound freedom. Nothing more.

But we're well aware that this dot-to-dot existence nestling in the gaps in our memories and consciousness won't satisfy us for long. It's not real life, not the one we aspire to. It's only a sham carpe diem, a compensatory recreation, a diversion. Someday it won't be enough. We'll want to take the blinders off the present and look the past and the future right in the eye. We'll want to remember and to project ourselves. Someday we'll want to live again, fully.

And so, slowly and patiently, we'll try to settle back into human time. It sure is a long, difficult apprenticeship for those who've survived disaster. It involves clambering up over the wreckage to find hope for the future. And, it turns out, it doesn't wait—it starts right now.

Little Hope

Once upon a time there was a little girl. A tiny little nothing of a girl. She was given plenty of names, by turns insignificant, comical, or miserable: flea, gnat, chopped ham, rug rat, kiddo, brat, minx, shitface, cling-on, pain. Even her given name—because, in spite of everything, she did have one—was proof of some shortcoming, because it was a diminutive of her mother's name. Deep down, however, everyone thought of her as "Little Hope."

Her birth was surrounded in mystery. She arrived by accident. But her mother had another version: she claimed she had conceived the child with a sort of mind-healer woman whom she saw three times a week. If she is to be believed, then, the child was the fruit of two women's minds, the one giving birth to the other once fertilized. Truth be told, it was an altogether peculiar story. A strange, maieutic tale that simultaneously robbed the child of a father and of flesh. Indeed, it would almost be enough to rob her of her existence too.

Begotten on a therapist's couch, Little Hope had to learn to grow up in its shadow. It was difficult to find space for herself because the urgent demands of the treatment quite filled the room. Absorbed by her not inconsiderable suffering, the mother was the sort to seek her own reflection in her newborn's eyes. She was the one who had had no father—hers had disappeared in an asylum. She was the one struggling to survive as best she could. She was the one putting all her strength into being reborn. To her the child was her mirror, her twin, her double in miniature. And therefore her diminutive. This child, then, must compensate for affection, siblings, family—all things of which she herself had been deprived. Must know to be there when she was needed and disappear when appropriate. This bestowed a very unusual status on Little Hope as she was not only invested with too much importance in her role but also rejected in herself. A pure projection, an orphan, empty and anonymous.

Nevertheless, there was a father. Alas, he too was woefully fragile. He had spent his youth in a suffocating home in the lunatic asylum where his parents worked. A place of impediments, emotional starvation, and unspoken secrets. Ever since, he had lived both in fear of and in service to this past. Like the shy people in Jacques Brel's song, he seemed to go through life with a suitcase in each hand. Guilt was his primary motivation. He had devoted himself to his wife's happiness as if he were indebted to her for something. Perhaps in this woman's domineering energy he found a strength that he himself lacked. And so he strove to spare her any displeasure, afraid that the least false move would puncture the powerful, vital, but unstable bubble they both so desperately needed. It was, in truth, a weighty burden feeling this never-ending need to satisfy, and it resulted in a constant gnawing tension that occasionally exploded cruelly. Hampered by too much heavy baggage and bundled up in his silence, the father would fly into violent rages, losing control of his actions and words.

Little Hope's birth constituted a safety valve in this overloaded system. When the pressure could no longer be contained, the child assumed her role as a substitute, at her father's tacit request. In her he could loathe with impunity all that he forbade himself despising in himself and his wife, without the risk of threatening their unstable status quo or of suffering any reprisals. He had nothing to fear from the child. She was defenseless. And so there were occasional humiliating acts—beating on a bare behind, cold showers on a hastily undressed body. More often than not, however, the blows were verbal. The child was branded intolerable and obnoxious. She had always ruined everything, had been in their way from the start, was unlovable. It was *just the way she was*. She need only look in the mirror and she would understand. The mother agreed wholeheartedly, even went further, escaping her own failings in this transfer of responsibility. Then the tension would drop as swiftly as it had escalated, and the parents would revert to a semblance of well-being thanks to the crisis. Referring back to it was strictly forbidden. The idea would not even have occurred to the child. She was familiar with their painful backgrounds and intuited unspeakable torments. And, on these grounds, forgave them. Perhaps she was also stunned by the sudden renewed calm after such storms. Her parents were once again refined, cultivated, subtle, sometimes funny, even loving. Touching. She, meanwhile, was back to being called an intelligent, easy, ever-smiling, inquisitive, receptive little girl, in other words, a dream child who was a pleasure to behold as the idyllic realization of family achievement. Little Hope.

Although not consciously, the child molded to fit this dysfunctional system. She developed a specific kind of sensitivity to it, aimed at identifying the first signs of an outburst. She was always on the alert, her senses vigilant, scrutinizing her parents for the precursors of an imminent catastrophe, careful to protect their universe from any potentially triggering factor. And so she went through her life like a sentinel, leaving behind her own self. The world around her she knew in great detail but of herself she knew very little. She simply made every effort, in both her actions and her words, not to cause any supplementary source of dissatisfaction. She never did anything wrong, did not lie, accepted instructions, anticipated orders, adapted to change, and stepped up to challenges. In everything she did—be it in the domestic sphere, leisure activities, sociability, or, most significantly, her schooling—she proved almost compulsorily sensible, gifted, and effectual. She was not aiming so much for perfection as for invisibility. And yet her efforts were in vain. Partly because she sometimes failed to not-be. Being playful and willful by nature, she always ended up disappointing with her overabundance of life. On these occasions she rebelled with scenes that were all the more capricious for having been kept in check so long, loaded with the injustice of her being held responsible for crises that were none of her doing, and feeding on the fear of initiating others. And this was because there were also many, many external elements liable to destabilize the delicate parental balance: bad weather, the cold, winter, Sundays, family, work, society, and all sorts of conditions about which Little Hope knew nothing. She was therefore always on her guard, monitoring her every footstep, her childhood warped because she was so completely everything and nothing in her parents' eyes.

She would have liked to have brothers and sisters to lean on, to build a rampart of childish nonchalance and complicity, to share times of happiness and perhaps also of sadness. She did in fact have three of them, three siblings. Two boys and a girl. But, being some ten years older, they had had a head start and constituted their own community with carefully concealed weaknesses. At first they said they would have preferred a dog, but it was not long before they realized that this was in fact better—Little Hope provided a solution to their problems. Surely collective tensions could be freely incarnated in this last offshoot that did not yet have any knowledge, the power of speech, or even a definitive form? It was too perfect a godsend and the process was already tried and tested. Frustration simply had to be transformed into aggression. Jealousy would serve as a driving force. After all, she was exasperating, this little thing with her unfailing good humor and her unconditional love, naively waiting for some reciprocation that no one was prepared to offer. She was exasperating because she was too affectionate, too clever, too sensitive, too everything. The truth was she was exasperating because she was, period. As in ancient civilizations, the group entrusted their collective survival to the sacrifice of a single individual. The conditions had been fulfilled: having arrived late, the child was elementally different to the community. She was immediately designated guilty, and better still she herself felt inherently guilty. And fundamentally illegitimate.

More often than not she was ignored. Her pleasures and pains were never mentioned unless to be mocked or belittled, and this indifference was the most exquisite torture. Nevertheless, her older siblings did sometimes come looking for her, when the need arose, one to dazzle by comparison, one to confide, another for distraction. She then ensured she was good company and an empathetic listener. Because she lived apart from them, she had grown accustomed to listening and watching, and could therefore guess at each of their private hurts—the exhausting quest for recognition in one, the emotional instability in another, and the failure complex in the third. She understood the causes of these hurts and forgave their consequences, despite the effect they had on her. Her siblings too were victims; they too were innocent. Like her parents, like herself. And yet she was wrong. The intimacy she felt in these shared exchanges was illusory. If Little Hope tried to talk about herself in return the others cut her short. Whatever cruel fate befell her, whatever injustice she felt, she always deserved it. In order to function properly, the mechanism needed to stay hidden. The others genuinely needed to believe she was at fault. And so they all forbade themselves to think about her for fear of having to admit the terrible truth. They couldn't run the risk of loving her.

This is how and why Little Hope felt like the custodian of a shameful secret that she herself did not know. It carved a hole in her heart. And yet she knew plenty of other hidden facts in this family. She even felt she was the only one to whom the buried traumas of the lineage had been passed down. The accidents, the illnesses, the mental problems, the grief. Guardian of these taboos, she now watched over the skeletons in the closets, behind her smile, like closed doors. In any given situation it was appropriate for her to hold her tongue and by doing this she allowed the essentials of her life to pass her by. She was not writing herself into her own story. And it was not the most significant incongruity of her childhood that she found she was both aware of everything and blind to herself.

Against all expectations, the family system was sustained when they reached adulthood. In this specific area,
the siblings never grew up. The discrepancies emerged.
Little Hope had a partner later, younger children, took a
different career, went to live in a different town, and even
in another country. She was not forgiven. The siblings lost
interest in her. They did not invite her to anything, did not
call her, did not come to see her. The family rarely got together in any event. Little Hope was reduced to being an
idea or a fantasy to her brothers and sisters. They knew
nothing about her. She continued to exist for them only
through their parents' words, words intended to keep her—
whether in admiration or criticism—in the separate place
that had been attributed to her from the start. She therefore
lost any chance of an objective existence and any possibility
of a meaningful relationship with her family.

One day an unusual tragedy struck Little Hope. One of
her children was diagnosed with a very serious illness. For
weeks, months, years she feared for his life. The violence
of the real world succeeded—for a time—in introducing
a chink in the system. The parents became parents, the
sister a sister. Only the brothers still wavered. The eldest
shut himself away in total avoidance, appearing only when
the treatment was over to celebrate this ending because, he

claimed, it had been intolerable, his mother couldn't talk about anything else. Jealousy made him omit the fact that this was by no means the end yet. The second brother hesitated and came to visit his nephew once but made a point of how much it cost him, financially. He and his wife had concluded that this illness was not in fact particularly serious and, at the end of the day, was preferable to the multiple operations endured by another nephew of theirs. The brothers agreed on this point, had discussed it, thereby ignoring not only the very real risk of death but also the poor taste of making the comparison. Besides, neither one of them thought to ask Little Hope how she was feeling. This indifference, far from being an abomination, actually proved liberating. It urged Little Hope to question her origins. When the illness was finally quashed, she asked her mother about the secrecy surrounding her birth. And in so doing found the keys to the mystery.

First of all there was a small piece of card, some three inches by four. Like an invitation or a greeting card. Or an announcement card. On it was a series of dates written in black ink, regularly, one under the other. Next to each date was an event, most of them sad. The signs needed deciphering. Cancers were noted with the initials "KC," deaths with a cross, anything else written out in full.

There were ten dates between 1967 and 1999, two cancers (Little Hope's father and grandfather), six deaths (her grandparents, her step-grandfather, and a great aunt), a fractured spine for her father, and surgery for her mother. Each person was identified by name or by their relationship to Little Hope's mother: her husband, her birth father, the stepfather who raised her, her mother, her aunt, etc. In 1971, huddled between a cancer and a death, came the birth of Little Hope. "It's not tragic," the mother said, "it's the map of a life." Little Hope simply wondered whose life she meant.

Her mother then handed her another element of her reply. A text to read, with no commentary. It was a poem by Charles Péguy called "A Little Hope," and it said:

> What surprises me, says God, is hope.
> I can't get over it.
> This little hope that looks like nothing at all.
> This little girl hope.
> Immortal hope.
> [. . .]
> Hope is a little nothing of a girl.
> [. . .]
> And yet this little girl will travel many worlds.
> This little nothing of a girl.
> She alone will carry the others as she travels long-lost
>   worlds.

[...]

Little hope walks between her two older sisters, and
goes quite unnoticed.

On the road to salvation and on the earthly path,
on the rocky path to salvation and on the never-
ending path, on the path between her sisters,
little hope

Keeps going.

Between her sisters.

One of them married.

The other a mother.

And all that anyone notices, all that Christian people
notice are the two older sisters.

[. . .]

One on the right and the other on the left.

And they hardly even see the girl in the middle.

The little one, who's still at school.

And who keeps walking.

Lost in her sisters' skirts.

And they readily believe that the older two are
leading the youngest along by the hand.

In the middle.

Between them.

To help her on this rocky path to salvation.

Only the blind cannot see the reverse.

That it's the child in the middle who's leading her
sisters.

And without her they would be nothing.
But two women already grown old.
Two elderly women.
Withered by life.

And she, the little one, leads them all.
[. . .]
Hope sees what has not yet been and what is to come.
She loves what has not yet been and what is to come.

In the future of time and of all eternity.

On that arduous, sandy, uphill path.
On the uphill road.
Dragged along, clinging to her sisters' arms,
As they hold her hand,
Little hope.
Keeps going.
And there, between her sisters, she appears to let
    them drag her.
Like a child too tired to walk.
Who might be hauled along this road in spite of
    herself.
When in fact she is the one getting the other two to
    walk.
And leading them along,
And moving the whole world forwards.

And leading it along.
Because no one ever works but for children.
And the older two would not walk but for little hope.

Little Hope folded up the poem again. She feigned naivete, claimed she did not understand why her mother was
showing it to her with its endless succession of theological al-
legories and emphatic pauses. She had been hoping for a more
candid answer. "Don't you think it's beautiful? It's magnificent. In fact, I sent it to everyone when you were born," her
mother told her with tears in her eyes. One feint deserves
another. "Well, I think it's kind of heavy-going," Little Hope
replied. "And I don't see what it has to do with me." She
certainly had no intention of discussing its aesthetics; this
was no literary soiree. Things needed saying, the system
clearly exposing, the mystery denouncing. Because, in truth,
she understood all too clearly what was being sought here,
intertextually—one last refuge. She had read every line of it,
had felt the effects of every word. Its anaphors, accumulations, parallelisms, amplifications and their downfalls, all its
rhetoric hammered into her soul the place that had instantly
been assigned to her before she was even born. Certainly not
the map of a life but a programmed intention. The messianic
child, sacrificed to collective redemption, both invisible and
essential, ignored and vital, everything and nothing. Nothing for being everything. Everything instead of being. She
felt like a dried butterfly, pinned on the white page of her

family's story. Inert, bloodless, frozen in a phantasmatic eternity. A sphinx-like skull stowed away in a box of secrets.

From then on it was all over with Little Hope. She would open the box, invent a new name for herself. She, for example. Or perhaps I. There was so much for this "I" to do. It would build itself slowly, patiently, bit by bit. It would write itself at length because before devoting herself to her own private remission, she had another to support. Not that of her family's sins but the far more real and tangible remission of her child's ailing body. The illness relinquishing its hold, the symptoms melting away, the period of observation, an interval of time during which hope of a recovery is born and grows and emerges. And with it the concomitant fear of a relapse. She knew the implications: the waiting, risks, anxieties, separations, and even potential grief. She also knew how hard it would be to pick out her own path in all this, with one foot in the cancer and one foot outside. It had to be survived. The child had to be completely saved, completely breaking away from his chrysalis, in order for her in turn to take flight. At least she could now envision making a start on her direction. "Right now," she told herself, "I'm the one who's going to hope."

Winter's here again. I can feel it in the crispness hitting my face, in the condensation I exhale and the distinctive tension in the air. But it's not the cold that strikes me, or the acute contrasts. Or even the almost metallic silence. It's a smell. An acrid, salty smell. It assaults my nostrils and seems to prickle my mucous surfaces. I don't recognize it at first. It doesn't belong here in the city, it's from somewhere else, somewhere far away, and yet it's very familiar. Eventually I get it: this smell isn't coming from outside, it's bubbling up from the depths of my body's memory. It's the smell of the hospital, the smell of the Institute. It came to me automatically by sensory association. My perception of winter triggered an olfactory memory of the Curie. Like a reflex. But this is not simply a question of reminiscence, this synesthesia produces a time loop, bringing the past trauma into the present and connecting it to the future. In a flash, before I'm even aware of the cold, my whole being has registered that winter is here, trailing behind it its retinue of unavoidable events like so many systematic consequences of this one imminent cause: It will soon be December 16. And on December 16 cancer strikes.

This icy morning is heralding a very strange anniversary indeed. It crystalizes the ambivalence of remission, a lull that could foreshadow fine days to come or a return to stormy weather. Fear of a relapse permanently torments the newfound freedom.

There has been a summer, though. Permission, at last, to leave Paris, a few days by the sea. The emotion of seeing our three children holding hands and running into the water. The eldest, you, looking bald, thin, and white with a scar under your armpit, and the younger two full of glee and energy; all of you rolling on the wet sand, throwing yourselves into the waves, grappling with each other. There were meals, games, laughs, fights, and the adoption of a cat. There was coming home in September and going back to school. There was even the regrowth of tiny little hairs here and there on your scalp. But there was also and there remains all the rest, all the aspects of lymphoma that still have a hold on you one way or another. You may be living your life but only under observation. There are many trips back to the Institute, every three weeks we have to check that the sleeping creature hasn't woken. Its hibernation carries no guarantees. You're asked to lie down on an examination bed in a small, dark room in the basement. Your neck, stomach, and groin are scanned. Outlines in black, gray, and white emerge on the screen, sound transformed into images. Dozens of tiny oval-shaped entities appear. They need be only slightly rounded, larger, or uniformly dark to attract more attention. Little black holes into which my mind topples. They are studied and measured, one by one. The silence is oppressive. The only talking is from the numbers appearing on the screen. Everyone knows that anything over half an inch means it could all start again. Breathing hangs on that fateful scale. Then it's back to see Dr. O on the sixth floor in the outpatient department. His clinical examination must confirm the findings of the ultrasound. It is punctuated at best with a "See you in three weeks." But the leave period is never actually that long; there are emergency consultations in the interim: with fear in our bellies we come back for an unexpected fever, worrying headaches, bloating in your stomach, a gland under your arm, a swelling tonsil. We also need to return here to treat the damage to our souls, yours and the whole family's. It has attacked in force, if somewhat delayed. When the body is no longer under fire, the mind is at war. And then a whole other fight begins, against trauma, against fear, against the world, against the self. A fight that can go on for years, until there is a complete recovery, and sometimes beyond. A fight that exhausts the individuals waging it, drives away friends, divides families, and breaks up couples.

No one comes out of the Institute unscathed. The truth is it's a struggle to get out of the place.

Of course, there's a longing to live and in the early stages everything is there to be rediscovered, the least thing is thrilling—the atmosphere of the outside world, the city's streets, starting school again, a family weekend, an evening with friends. Returning to normal life is a giddying surprise, even routine is in itself a wonderful break. But soon people find this isn't enough, they hanker for more, to make up for lost time. Time given over to the illness and before that too.

*And so they invent new possibilities, they quiver with enthu-
siasm, jealously guard their freedom, and, in everything they
do, they aspire to the essence of life. They find themselves
dreaming of untried pleasures and unfulfilled desires, of ex-
tensive travels and boundless love. They consume existence
avidly, voraciously. With bulimic intensity.*

*At the same time they find it difficult to get anywhere,
they feel hampered, as if they've forgotten how to live. This
is because they're still so weighed down with what they've just
been through, wearing their trauma on their sleeve. Simply because it has happened once means the accident is now always
possible. And so each of them individually blunders forward,
doubly burdened by a painful past and a worrying future. It's
a heavy load and it gives them a halting step.*

*By its very nature, lymphoma exaggerates these paradoxes
of remission. Its invisibility is the first reason for this: it's not
the sort to leave evidence of its visit. It's a sneaky, insidious
enemy, an internal enemy. It likes to pillage without leaving a
trace and to drain without obvious damage. No flesh, organs,
or bones are vandalized. There's no operation, enucleation,
or amputation. Nothing seems to be missing from the body it
has affected. Not even a modest tonsil. With this performance
it's easy to assume the danger is over, but this wholeness is
only superficial. Lymphoma doesn't appear in any one place
because it can potentially strike anywhere. It's never where it's
expected to be and doesn't show up in the same place twice. It
acts like a terrorist, preparing its attacks in secret and striking*

blind, so that no one can be entirely reassured when it's no longer there to see. This might even be more worrying. People therefore come to dread this sleeping threat that lies low, always ready to loom back out of the shadows like a big cat releasing its prey to get a better hold of it. They hesitate to make the most of what may be a false deliverance, intended specifically to make a future reconquest all the more delectable. Perfidious lymphoma, a despicable traitor that leaves its victims with their arms and legs in order to become a phantom limb of the whole body. It will never stop making them suffer. Even its absence is a painful presence. And added to this is the remarkable speed of its development at every stage. It certainly germinates and propagates itself far more quickly than it beats a retreat. An acute emergency, doubling in volume every twelve hours, it invades the body in the space of a few days, when months can be spent overwhelming its first attacks. But the chemotherapy campaign, which feels never-ending to the patient and his or her family, turns out to be relatively short on a scale of other oncological treatments. Lymphoma drags its victims into its tormented world, imposing a breakneck tempo on them so that they lose all their bearings. It raids them violently for no apparent reason and then suddenly drops them with no more explanation. Even in the jaws of defeat it still puts pressure on them. Everything happens too quickly; how can anyone feel safe afterward? How can they fail to dread another onslaught from such a summarily destructive force? They're traumatized.

Paris, year zero. On the ruins of the old world everything needs rebuilding. It's not easy conceiving the new architecture. Good, solid foundations need digging out, the sort that can withstand any assault. In this devastated city a child battles to become a child again. To learn to play again, and rediscover his innocence. To learn to learn again. He asks the adults around him for help and, whatever their own wounds, they cannot let him down now. They've protected this child through the bleakest hours and must now protect him from the woes of the postwar period. That metaphor may be overused but what does it matter? People can call the thing whatever they like—in all its horror, it deserves no better. I would not forgive myself if I tried to find pretty names for it or dressed it up in fine words or opened wide the door to the imagination for it. So why not use martial images? It could just as easily be natural ones: this blitz, this cataclysm with the enemy variously identified as a tsunami, a landslide, an earthquake, a tornado, a cyclone, or a flood. And why not cosmic? Asteroids, meteorites, black holes? A big bang, while we're at it. But that's how it goes with metaphors, they stick. They have a tough life. Martial they have been and martial they'll remain. It doesn't change anything, anyway. Desolation goes by only one name. The wreckage is still wreckage and the victims are still victims. And so everyone takes up arms once more. Full of courage, optimism, drive, and patience. And most of all hope.

———

Here we all are, then—you, your brother and sister, and the two of us, all intoxicated by remission, disabled adventurers ready to reconquer the world in our own limping way. It's a long journey. First, we need to break away from the Institute, and this doesn't mean simply forgetting medical checks, which take us back there regularly, but also gradually unraveling the emotional ties that bind us to it. Because this place, originally so alien and hostile, has become extraordinarily familiar. Over the months we learned its language, molded to its codes, and adopted its customs. We ended up liking this world and its inhabitants. Together we wrote a story. Sick children, parents, and loved ones were our equals, our brothers in arms; caregivers, administrators, and technicians our allies. We had no choice. Now, though, it feels as if we must unlearn the very things that have helped anchor us if we are to recover aspects of our lives from which we so painfully abdicated. Reliving in reverse the highs and lows of the beginning, redefining our here and our there once more, reinverting our values, retracing our steps in the opposite direction. We're like exiles who return to their homeland after a long absence: everyone agrees it's a difficult experience and involves many challenges. As if returning from exile, then, it won't be easy for us to get our bearings. As if returning from exile, we'll find it hard to integrate. As if returning from exile, we'll have to explore our identity in order to rebuild a home.

That's what it's like coming out of the Institute: everything's still there but nothing's exactly as before. Neither completely the same nor completely different. An indefinable difference hovers over everything. It's not so much about places, which are relatively unchanging, but about people. The streets are still where they've always been, buildings stand in their usual places, and shops have their regular frontage. At the very most the neighborhood seems particularly lively. People, on the other hand, present an unexpected picture. Where we might have hoped for, if not a celebration of your return, at least a warm welcome, a complex social fabric is woven.

At school, for a start. "Your cancer changed you too much," say some of your friends who'd rather not be friends anymore. Out of fear or shyness, tactlessness, or jealousy for the attention given in absentia to this friend with the different story, when they feel ignored in their own struggles—divorcing parents, siblings torn apart, academic failure, loneliness, and other private childhood dramas. "I'd really like to play with you," say others who, by contrast, weren't close before but would now like to be your friends. Out of empathy or pity, curiosity or exceptional maturity fueled by the experience of some unspoken trauma. New friendships emerge and, without actually healing the wound, they compensate for the affections lost. In their own way, these friendships too are now the bastard children of cancer. Even after it has been eradicated the enemy continues, in good ways and in bad, to subject children's relationships to its evil laws.

Adults don't appear to be any freer, also bowing to the enemy's yolk to a greater or lesser extent. "I'm no longer talking to you. You didn't come to my birthday even though I'd hurt my foot. All you could think about was your son," one woman says in front of the friendly group gathered at the local café. The others, stunned, don't intervene. They look away and, showing no reaction, descend into the cowardice of collaborators bankrolled by some armchair philosophy. After all, it has to be said, we all have our problems. The bar's still here, the percolator's purring, the regulars are drinking, but the Café d'Avant, the "Before Café," has gone. "We've had enough of this cancer business. It's like a bad smell in the neighborhood. We just want an easy life," someone else tells your sister at the end of school, and she forbids her daughter to talk to Anna anymore. Two little girls in tears, yet more collateral victims. Even the family don't escape its clutches: "We're glad it's over. It's all Mom could talk about," says someone else, my brother, as we know. In your maternal and paternal families the page is turned in the same way, in silence. Widespread indifference. They don't put on parties for your homecoming or celebrate your courage. They don't all head off on vacation together with us. They pretend they didn't see anything. There won't be a single glass drunk to your health, not a single wink or a single word. For some adults—whether

they are more or less battle-hardened, brave, or empathetic—this is their way of submitting to the diktats of fear,
without even thinking about it, and they draw a pretense
of strength from their least noble resources: resentment, ri-
valry, pettiness, naivete, stupidity, and selfishness. Their
small-minded settling of accounts with fate, set against the
background of their schoolyard mentality.

And this goes on for months, years. It goes on long after
the last visible signs of the illness have faded away. Social
rehabilitation definitely doesn't proceed at the same rate as
physical recovery. It's still way behind when you're already
looking as you used to. In fact, your face and body quickly
achieve a healthy shape and color. The one deflating, the
other gaining in size. In the end you do look quite like you
did before. Particularly as the chemotherapy arrested your
growth; you haven't grown even half an inch since you went
into the hospital. In some ways you look more like yourself now because your hair, which is growing back black
with very tight curls, now testifies to your origins. Along
with the soft tan of our few days by the sea, it makes you
look like a real Tunisian. Apart from your discreet scars—
reminders of your implanted port-a-cath—the lymphoma
left no marks on you. Only your nails now bear subtle witness to it: every one of them has a series of stripes parallel to
the lunula. These lines are like watermarks, implicit signs
of repeated stops in nail growth because of treatments. A
trained eye could read the story of your battle in these white

tracks, like deciphering the age of a tree from the rings in its trunk. But there are few trained eyes; to the world in general, everything looks normal.

As for the rest of us, I don't know whether we bear visible signs of our ordeal. No one mentions them, in any event; we're spared that. I would have thought it could be gauged in the pallor of our skin, the depth of our wrinkles, and the sagging of our features. I don't waste much time on this. Only the three white hairs that have sprouted incongruously amid your little brother's childish curls seem to me to be secret manifestations of how your family shared in your suffering. Those hairs will never be brown again. We have all aged, for sure. Does it really not show? Now that I think about it, I do think I can make out a trace of it in your eyes. They're deeper, more serious, and more intense than before.

Maybe, Lise thinks, that's where it can be found, this indefinable difference. Not so much in things and people but the expressions in people's eyes. The way the world looks at them and the way they look at the world.

On the one hand they need to reconstitute their identity in other people's eyes, to become more than the sick child, the brother or sister of the sick child, and the father or mother of the sick child. It's no mean feat. The family seems to lug lymphoma around like some cursed legacy. It's an invisible canker, an ulceration of the soul that some people are afraid of catching. The family's very presence displays the unendurable and screams the unutterable. Because they have rubbed shoulders with the truth they are now abominable in the eyes of the world, forcing others to see what they don't want to see, hear what they don't want to hear, and think what they don't want to think. Pushing the boundaries of their defenses and driving them toward the abyss. This explains, if not forgives, all the apathy, the exclusions, and the lost friendships. How can they resent this? People's injustice quite naturally makes its bed on the injustices of life. In most cases, this is simply for protection, but for the patients and their families it is a double punishment. It pains Solal terribly; he says that these rejections are harder blows to bear than the illness. Knowing he's confronted with this new ordeal drives his mother mad, makes her want to rebel. She doesn't know what to say to him, couldn't justify the fact that, in some people's eyes, they themselves have become this terrible cancer. In spite of themselves, but just as obscene and monstrous.

Branded as different, they now find it's impossible to view life in the same way as before. Their reality has been refracted through the prism of lymphoma. Nothing is straight or reliable now. Not relationships, certainties, loyalties, expectations, or plans. All of them jagged, refracted lines. Of course they know what would be the right thing to do: to throw themselves wholeheartedly into life, embracing the present and denying the elements of cancer that still haunt them. Pretending. Pretending *they don't know. Pretending they haven't seen. Pretending it's all over. It's a wasted effort. No one can plead ignorance to him- or herself. They long to and strive to all the same. And now here they are masquerading as the Anybody family, laughing at the same jokes, enjoying the same pastimes, and responding indignantly to the same trifles. Their social identity is forged through successive acts of anonymity. They even force themselves to forget; they'd do anything to belong to the world of the living again. With time, this silent insistence on being happy proves even worse than feeling different. It brings with it a sort of moral denial, in which they feel they're losing their way. And yet they serve it up to themselves more than others serve it up to them. Only the Institute seems to save them from sliding off course. Here everyone knows and here they're allowed to be not 100 percent happy. Not straightaway, at least. It might be a psychologist helping them gently toward an "after." A nurse giving them a hug, moved by what they've been through. Or a secretary telling them confidentially about other parents' struggles even years after a recovery. It's a whole world of its own in which they can, to some extent, recognize themselves again. Both the same and different. As they are inside, irrevocably changed.*

Then the time comes for the whys. Some of which can be resolved and others that remain unanswered. And the latter kind need chewing over at length. Then they feel guilty. Guilty for not anticipating, not guessing. Guilty for not protecting. Even perhaps guilty for causing.

It will take many years to accept that they simply saw the world as it is.

And then. And then there are the others. The ones who stayed at the Institute and, worse still, those who'll never leave. The little girl with the scar over her head. The teenager with the empty sleeve. Marion who will never grow into a woman. Dense ghosts whose absence weighs heavy and haunts us. We have to cope with them, or rather without them. Without even realizing we're experiencing survivor guilt. Barely a few days by the sea and you're having nightmares about it already. You see yourself on a beautiful island with your family around you and on the mainland nearby is an isolated prison from which you've just escaped. To get to us you got past a huge wall erected halfway across the sea. You couldn't have climbed it; you went under it. You had to dive deep into the cold black waters. You had to hold your breath, for a long time. You almost drowned, several times, but you made it. Blind and starved of oxygen, you got away. We welcomed you on the shore and we're so happy to be together. We're happily celebrating our reunion when we hear cries coming from the far side of the wall. You can see dozens of children there, your former fellow sufferers. They haven't managed to escape. Some have gone back to the mainland, disheartened, others are still struggling, but with no success. Still others float on their stomachs, their arms out in a cross shape and their faces submerged. Your find their inert bodies even more frightening than the captives' calls. You wake sweating and crying.

There's one person in particular, a twenty-year-old musician, a radiant, elegant young man called Gabriel. The son of a very dear friend. Pierre's son. He was diagnosed shortly after you were, treated at the same time as you, in another hospital and for a different cancer. Fatal in his case. A sickening coincidence in which our fates as unlucky parents at first converged before diverging in terror while our friendship forged its means of resistance. We'll have to cope without that boy too. Later, at almost the same time, we'll write books—Pierre's about his son's death and mine about your survival. My friend will have confronted the worst form of grief while I will only have buried a ghost. Beside him I'll feel illegitimate and ridiculous, both in my suffering and in my words. Pierre will give me a copy of his book three days before it's published, three days before I finish writing mine. I won't read it straightaway. It will be named after a piece composed by Gabriel, *Winter Is Coming.*

Oh yes, winter will just keep on coming back.

———

A long, long time ago, well before history and books existed, people lived on earth free of sorrow, hard work, and cruel sickness. Or so the poet says.

Humans were weak, though. Naked and defenseless to confront the other creatures. Among the immortals there was a rebellious spirit prepared to embrace their cause. In order to teach them the ways of art and science, he offered humans the sacred fire, stolen from the gods. This displeased the supreme master, the father of the gods and of men, who reigned over celestial spheres, and he decided to take revenge. Using clay and water, he fashioned a woman and bestowed every gift on her. He offered her in marriage to the rebel's brother. The woman carried a mysterious earthenware urn that she had been advised to keep closed. This urn alone contained all the ills of humankind— old age, famine, madness, war, vice, passion, pride, and hope. Being inquisitive by nature, the woman couldn't resist lifting the lid. The ills escaped and spread far and wide. Only hope stayed in the urn. Waiting on the lip of the receptacle, it did not fly free before the lid was replaced. Ever since that day, a thousand calamities have assailed humankind from every direction. The earth is full of plagues and the sea is full of them too; diseases delight in tormenting mortals day and night, silently dealing out every kind of agony. Or so the poet says.

It is indeed a strange thing, this hope hidden away in the bottom of the urn, like a secret in its box. Unable to escape, too slow or too inept, it seems to be trailing a foot, perhaps it is lame. Even its name is unattractive: it is called Elpis, a *funny name with unfortunate, slightly ridiculous resonances to modern ears. It is like a child's word, and is almost inappropriate for such an imposing concept. And anyway, what's it doing in this urn, in among all these creatures with their dark intentions? Its very presence poses questions. Is disturbing. Which is why some wish the story were different. They wish the urn were filled not with ills but with wonders and that, once these have escaped, hope remains to console mankind for this loss. History can always be rewritten. And yet this does nothing to erase previous versions. What was said is said. What was thought is perpetuated. The hesitation is still there. The enigma unresolved.*

Perhaps when all is said and done that's what hope is. Not the certainty of a happy future, which is the prerogative of the immortals. Nor dumb ignorance of the inevitable, the privilege of animals. But the tense, awkward, tortuous waiting between fear and the act of hoping in the face of an uncertain future. Waiting as someone who both knows and doesn't know. Everything encapsulated in it: confidence and terror, good and evil, the best and the worst, life and death, all inseparable characteristics of Elpis. With the lid back down, it hoards them all in its box of secrets. This Elpis is no little hope; it is measured. It isn't perfect; it's one-eyed. It isn't accompanied; it travels alone. It needs no one and trawls no one along with it. And yet it isn't singular; it's plural. It carries so many hopes within it. Laden with these hopes, it travels its difficult path, clearly and resolutely accepting what is to come.

Spring 2015

Once we're back home, music reclaims its rights and a song is written on the ruins of the months that have trickled by. It comes from far, far away. From a note repeated endlessly in the void. An A. The A of a drip pump.

The song is called "Big Bang" and describes how your world exploded, how chaos proliferated, everything was atomized, and then new life breathed into us. That A forms an obstinate baseline, beating out the rhythm. In the middle of the song the voice is silent and the only thing is that A, inhabiting the silence and giving a sound-shape to what can't be said.

You're here. I'm not making it up. You really are here. Freed from the Institute and its machines with their gloomy notes. And so I sing in order to forget, to forget the risks you still run, forget my fear, forget uncertainty. Yes, Solal, we must sing, we must keep singing obstinately.

But even so, what if? What if?

In spite of everything, there's always an if.